PULMONARY AND RESPIRATORY DISEASES AND DISORDERS

INTERSTITIAL LUNG DISEASE

CAUSES, DIAGNOSIS AND TREATMENT

PULMONARY AND RESPIRATORY DISEASES AND DISORDERS

Additional books and e-books in this series can be found on Nova's website under the Series tab.

PULMONARY AND RESPIRATORY DISEASES AND DISORDERS

INTERSTITIAL LUNG DISEASE

CAUSES, DIAGNOSIS AND TREATMENT

LIVA T. VILLADSEN
EDITOR

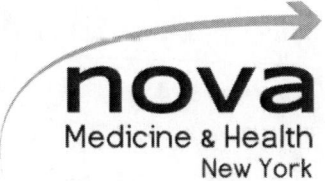

Copyright © 2019 by Nova Science Publishers, Inc.

All rights reserved. No part of this book may be reproduced, stored in a retrieval system or transmitted in any form or by any means: electronic, electrostatic, magnetic, tape, mechanical photocopying, recording or otherwise without the written permission of the Publisher.

We have partnered with Copyright Clearance Center to make it easy for you to obtain permissions to reuse content from this publication. Simply navigate to this publication's page on Nova's website and locate the "Get Permission" button below the title description. This button is linked directly to the title's permission page on copyright.com. Alternatively, you can visit copyright.com and search by title, ISBN, or ISSN.

For further questions about using the service on copyright.com, please contact:
Copyright Clearance Center
Phone: +1-(978) 750-8400　　　　Fax: +1-(978) 750-4470　　　　E-mail: info@copyright.com.

NOTICE TO THE READER

The Publisher has taken reasonable care in the preparation of this book, but makes no expressed or implied warranty of any kind and assumes no responsibility for any errors or omissions. No liability is assumed for incidental or consequential damages in connection with or arising out of information contained in this book. The Publisher shall not be liable for any special, consequential, or exemplary damages resulting, in whole or in part, from the readers' use of, or reliance upon, this material. Any parts of this book based on government reports are so indicated and copyright is claimed for those parts to the extent applicable to compilations of such works.

Independent verification should be sought for any data, advice or recommendations contained in this book. In addition, no responsibility is assumed by the Publisher for any injury and/or damage to persons or property arising from any methods, products, instructions, ideas or otherwise contained in this publication.

This publication is designed to provide accurate and authoritative information with regard to the subject matter covered herein. It is sold with the clear understanding that the Publisher is not engaged in rendering legal or any other professional services. If legal or any other expert assistance is required, the services of a competent person should be sought. FROM A DECLARATION OF PARTICIPANTS JOINTLY ADOPTED BY A COMMITTEE OF THE AMERICAN BAR ASSOCIATION AND A COMMITTEE OF PUBLISHERS.

Additional color graphics may be available in the e-book version of this book.

Library of Congress Cataloging-in-Publication Data

ISBN: 978-1-53616-246-2

Published by Nova Science Publishers, Inc. † New York

CONTENTS

Preface		vii
Chapter 1	Genetics in Interstitial Lung Diseases *Malay Sarkar and Smriti Mishra*	1
Chapter 2	Imaging of Acute Infiltrative Lung Disease *Meriem Affes, Henda Nèji, Monia Attia, Saoussen Hantous-Zannad, Ines Baccouche, Jammoussi Amira and Khaoula Ben Miled-M'rad*	75
Chapter 3	Imaging of Idiopathic and Connectivitis- Associated Interstitial Pneumonias *Monia Attia, Mariem Affes, Henda Nèji, Houda Gharsalli, Ines Baccouche*	113
Chapter 4	Lung Sarcoidosis: Typical and Atypical Features on Computed Tomography *Henda Nèji, Monia Attia, Mariem Affes, Houda Gharsalli, Ines Baccouche, Khaoula Ben Miled-M'rad and Saoussen Hantous-Zannad*	141

| **Chapter 5** | Cardio-Pulmonary Treatment in Systemic Sclerosis Patients: A Clinical Guide
Roberto G Carbone, Assaf Monselise and Francesco Puppo | **161** |

Index **185**

Related Nova Publications **189**

PREFACE

Interstitial lung diseases are a diverse group of acute and chronic pulmonary disorders characterized by a variable amount of inflammation and/or fibrosis. In Interstitial Lung Disease: Causes, Diagnosis and Treatment, the authors explore the role of genetics in the pathogenesis of interstitial lung diseases, as well as develop new diagnostic modalities and identify novel therapeutic targets.

This compilation goes on to discuss acute infiltrative lung disease, a heterogeneous group of lung disorders characterized by diffuse parenchymal lung involvement. This group of infiltrative lung diseases may result in five histopathological presentations: diffuse alveolar damage, diffuse alveolar hemorrhage, immunoallergic pneumonia, acute organizing pneumonia and acute eosinophilic pneumonia.

High-resolution computed tomography is proposed as a more sensitive and accurate method in diagnosing interstitial lung disease through specific patterns which are highly suggestive of a subtype of interstitial pneumonia.

High-resolution computed tomography is also proposed for the diagnosis of sarcoidosis, a systemic granulomatous disease which involves the lungs in more than 90% of cases. It is one of the leading causes of interstitial involvement in lung diseases, and its diagnosis is based on compatible clinical, biological, imaging and anatomopathological features.

The closing chapter aims to identify diagnostic procedures for the early diagnosis of cardio-pulmonary complications, delineate a proper methodology to monitor complications, and define therapeutic guidelines.

Chapter 1 - Interstitial lung diseases (ILDs) are a diverse group of ~200 acute and chronic pulmonary disorders characterized by a variable amount of inflammation and/or fibrosis. The ILDs of unknown aetiology are known as idiopathic interstitial pneumonia (IIP) and idiopathic pulmonary fibrosis (IPF) is the most common type of IIP. Other causes include collagen vascular disease, granulomatous ILDs, and environmental and drug exposure. These diseases are associated with substantial morbidity and mortality. The median survival of IPF is only two to five years. Misdiagnosis or delayed diagnosis is not uncommon which may lead to poor prognosis. Credible evidences are available suggesting that ILDs are caused by the gene-environment interactions. Studies have indicated the significant roles of genetic alterations of disease candidate genes in association with miRNAs and/or SNPs in ILDs pathogenesis. Several disease-associated rare and common genetic variants have been identified in both, familial and sporadic IPF cases. These genetic loci are involved in different biological processes, including alveolar stability, host defence, cell–cell barrier function, and cell senescence. These genetic variants play an important role in disease causation, progression of ILD, pharmacogenomics phenotyping and outcome. The knowledge of the roles of genetics will help us in understanding the pathogenesis, developing new diagnostic modalities and identifying novel therapeutic targets in future.

Chapter 2 - Acute infiltrative lung disease (AILD) is a heterogeneous group of lung disorders characterized by diffuse parenchymal lung involvement. It consists of an infiltrate of the interstitial lung tissue and/or distal airways (alveoli and respiratory bronchioles) which mainly occurs within 2 weeks and does not exceed one month. This group of infiltrative lung diseases may correspond to five histopathological presentations: diffuse alveolar damage, diffuse alveolar hemorrhage, immunoallergic pneumonia, acute organizing pneumonia and acute eosinophilic pneumonia. Each nosological entity may result from several causes. Moreover, the same disorder may have different histopathological manifestations.

AILD may result from many conditions. The main pathological causes are infections (bacterial, viral, fungal or parasitic) and hemodynamic overload (left ventricular failure). Cardiogenic pulmonary edema is easily suggested in the majority of cases on a chest CT scan. Typically, it is made up of regular septal thickening, "ground glass" opacities and consolidations associated with cardiomegaly, left atrium and pulmonary vein enlargement. Infections could be suggested in particular clinical conditions associated with *biologic inflammatory syndrome*. A bronchoalveolar lavage (BAL) is very useful, in this case, for the etiological diagnosis (pneumocystis, viruses...).

In addition to these common conditions, other rare causes have to be considered: acute respiratory distress syndrome, acute hypersensitivity pneumonitis, exposure to toxic gases and drugs including heroin or cocaine, connective tissue disease, or vasculitis which most often presents with alveolar hemorrhage. Acute Idiopathic organized pneumonia and acute idiopathic eosinophilic pneumonia are exclusion diagnoses.

A chest CT scan remains an essential examination in the assessment of AILD. A surgical pulmonary biopsy is unusual in the acute context. First of all, CT is useful in choosing the most suitable site for the BAL. It can suggest the cause in many cases. Semiological analysis of elementary lesions should be integrated with clinical data and the results of the BAL. There are different elementary patterns of AILD on CT scans including "ground glass" opacities, consolidations, septal thickening and micronodules. Their distribution as well as the predominant elementary lesions are helpful for diagnosis.

Chapter 3 - Interstitial pneumonias are a group of heterogeneous lung diseases that may be idiopathic or associated with an underlying abnormality such as connectivitis.

Imaging plays an essential role in characterizing this group of disorders and can often help identify the diagnosis.

A chest X-ray is often the first examination to suggest lung interstitial involvement.

However, it provides only limited information and is primarily used to rule out a differential diagnosis, such as left heart failure.

High-resolution computed tomography (HRCT) is more sensitive and accurate in diagnosing interstitial lung disease.

It plays a central role in recognizing and classifying this group of diseases through specific CT features and patterns which are highly suggestive of a subtype of interstitial pneumonia.

However, many of them share common imaging characteristics with significant overlap.

HRCT aims to find associated signs which may lead to suspicions of an associated connective tissue disease. It also allows a patient's prognosis to be evaluated and followed up with.

Although HR-CT is a cornerstone of an interstitial pneumonia diagnosis, a multidisciplinary approach is mandatory to best manage the patient.

Chapter 4 - Sarcoidosis is a systemic granulomatous disease which involves the lungs in more than 90% of cases. It is one of the leading causes of interstitial involvement in lung diseases. Its diagnosis is based on compatible clinical, biological, imaging and anatomopathological features. Thus, imaging is considered to be a cornerstone in the work-up and follow-up of the disease. High-resolution computed tomography (HR-CT) is more sensitive and more accurate than plain chest radiography in diagnosing parenchymal involvement.

In the inflammatory active forms, CT, typically shows micronodules of perilymphatic distribution, involving, the bronchovascular bundle, interlobular septa and fissures. In the fibrotic forms, patients present with one of three different patterns: bronchial distortion with or without central pseudo-masses, honeycombing or an irregular linear pattern. Classically, all these features are bilateral, symmetric, and involve the upper, mid and posterior parts of the lungs.

Atypical presentations include nodules and masses with irregular margins, alveolar consolidations, excavations, ground glass opacities, predominant septal thickening, miliary appearance, large and small airways involvement with air trapping. Features may be also distributed in an atypical manner to one side or to the lower parts of the lungs.

Radiological diagnosis is often easy in typical forms but may be challenging in some cases. Excluding lung cancer, carcinomatous lymphangitis and necrotizing as well as mycobacterial infections may sometimes be necessary.

Chapter 5 - About 10-15 percent of Systemic sclerosis (SSc) patients develop severe lung disease, which presents in two forms: a) pulmonary fibrosis (hardening or scarring of lung tissue because of collagen excess), b) pulmonary arterial hypertension (high blood pressure in the artery that carries blood from the heart to the lungs). Treatment for these two conditions is different. Pulmonary fibrosis may be treated with immunosuppressive drugs associated with low doses of corticosteroids, while pulmonary arterial hypertension (PAH) may be treated with drugs that dilate blood vessels such as prostacyclin. In order to improve quality of life (QOL) and prognosis of SSc patients, early diagnosis of cardio-pulmonary complications and a proper therapeutic approach are required. Aims of this chapter are to: 1) identify diagnostic procedures for early diagnosis of cardio-pulmonary complications; 2) delineate a proper methodology to monitor complications; 3) define therapeutic guidelines.

In: Interstitial Lung Disease
Editor: Liva T. Villadsen

ISBN: 978-1-53616-246-2
© 2019 Nova Science Publishers, Inc.

Chapter 1

GENETICS IN INTERSTITIAL LUNG DISEASES

Malay Sarkar[1,], MD and Smriti Mishra[2], PhD Scholar*
[1]Department of Pulmonary Medicine,
Indira Gandhi Medical College,
Shimla, Himachal Pradesh, India
[2]Department of Biotechnology and Bioinformatics,
Jaypee University of Information Technology,
Waknaghat, Solan, Himachal Pradesh, India

ABSTRACT

Interstitial lung diseases (ILDs) are a diverse group of ~200 acute and chronic pulmonary disorders characterized by a variable amount of inflammation and/or fibrosis. The ILDs of unknown aetiology are known as idiopathic interstitial pneumonia (IIP) and idiopathic pulmonary fibrosis (IPF) is the most common type of IIP. Other causes include collagen vascular disease, granulomatous ILDs, and environmental and drug exposure. These diseases are associated with substantial morbidity and mortality. The median survival of IPF is only two to five years.

---

* Corresponding Author's Email: drsarkarmalay23@rediffmail.com.

Misdiagnosis or delayed diagnosis is not uncommon which may lead to poor prognosis. Credible evidences are available suggesting that ILDs are caused by the gene-environment interactions. Studies have indicated the significant roles of genetic alterations of disease candidate genes in association with miRNAs and/or SNPs in ILDs pathogenesis. Several disease-associated rare and common genetic variants have been identified in both, familial and sporadic IPF cases. These genetic loci are involved in different biological processes, including alveolar stability, host defence, cell–cell barrier function, and cell senescence. These genetic variants play an important role in disease causation, progression of ILD, pharmacogenomics phenotyping and outcome. The knowledge of the roles of genetics will help us in understanding the pathogenesis, developing new diagnostic modalities and identifying novel therapeutic targets in future.

Keywords: familial pulmonary fibrosis, mucin, surfactant, telomere, telomerase, TOLLIP

1. INTRODUCTION

Interstitial lung disease (ILD) is a heterogeneous group of diffuse parenchymal lung disorders and is characterised by varying degrees of damage to the lung parenchyma via inflammation and fibrosis [1]. Apart from the interstitium, ILD also involves the airspaces, peripheral airways, and vessels along with their respective epithelial and endothelial linings. There are more than 200 different lung disorders listed under the umbrella term ILD that display considerable variation in terms of clinical course, treatment, and prognosis [2, 3] and the diagnosis of ILD is based on the combination of clinical, radiological, and histopathologic features. Types of ILD include idiopathic interstitial pneumonia (IIP) and ILD with identifiable causes, such as environmental exposure, drugs, tobacco smoke, genetic disorders, and autoimmune diseases. Idiopathic pulmonary fibrosis (IPF) is one of the most common types of ILD and is seen in approximately 50% of patients with IIP [4]. IPF is a chronic, progressive, fibrosing interstitial pneumonia of unknown aetiology that mainly occurs in older adults and is associated with a radiological and/or histopathological pattern of usual interstitial pneumonia (UIP) [5]. IPF is a prototype example of progressive-fibrosing ILD with a median survival of two to five years [6].

ILD is caused by interactions between genes and environmental factors [7] and a candidate-gene approach, genome-wide association studies (GWAS), and whole exome sequencing have been helpful in enhancing the understanding of the genetic origins of ILD. There is considerable variability in the development of the disease among individuals with exposure to similar concentrations of fibrogenic dusts or organic antigens and not all patients with exposure to asbestos or bleomycin or with a smoking history develop pulmonary fibrosis, indicating a genetic component of the disease [8, 9]. Pulmonary fibrosis has also been reported in association with many rare genetic disorders, such as dyskeratosis congenita (DC) [10], Hermansky-Pudlak syndrome [11], familial hypercalcaemic hypocalciuria [12], neurofibromatosis [13], tuberous sclerosis [14], and Gaucher disease [15] and among closely related family members. Indeed, familial clustering of pulmonary fibrosis cases has been reported in the literature for many years and is the most compelling epidemiological evidence for a genetic basis of pulmonary fibrosis. The first report of familial IPF was published in 1907 by Sandoz [16]. Familial clustering has been reported in various settings: monozygotic twins lived in different environments [17, 18, 19] consecutive generations in the same families [19, 20, 21] and family members separated at an early age [22]. The role of genetics in ILD is an evolving one, however, it has the potential to improve early diagnosis, the assessment of patient response to therapy, and prognostication. This chapter will therefore focus on the role of various genes in ILD.

2. GENETIC VARIANTS

Several common and rare genetic variants have been identified in patients with both sporadic and familial forms of pulmonary fibrosis. Common variants are defined by a minor allele frequency (MAF) of more than 5%, whereas rare variants have an MAF of less than 0.1% [23]. There are four broad categories of the biological processes controlled by the genes implicated in ILD development: alveolar stability; host defence; cell-cell barrier function; and cell senescence [23].

3. GENOME-WIDE ASSOCIATION STUDY (GWAS)

Candidate gene approaches and GWAS are the two most common genetic methods for identifying the susceptibility variants and the latter have identified several genetic loci associated with a susceptibility to IPF [24]. In a GWAS including 159 IPF patients and 934 controls with replication analysis in 83 cases and 535 controls, Mushiroda et al. found a significant association between single nucleotide polymorphisms (SNP) *rs2736100* in intron 2 of the telomerase reverse transcriptase *(TERT)* gene and IPF risk [25]. This SNP is located within a linkage disequilibrium (LD) block in the *TERT* gene, indicating that *rs2736100* may have been associated with another unidentified variation within *TERT* in this Japanese cohort of IPF patients. This was the first common variant associated with sporadic IPF in the Japanese population to be confirmed by GWAS and two landmark GWAS were performed in both familial and sporadic IPF patients in 2013 that identified several SNPs within a number of loci that suggested susceptibility to pulmonary fibrosis [26, 27].

Fingerlin et al. performed a GWAS of 1,616 non-Hispanic, White individuals with fibrotic IIPs and 4,683 controls with follow-up replication analyses in 876 cases and 1,890 controls [26]. The majority of the IIP cases had a diagnosis of IPF. Besides confirming the known associations with *TERT* at 5p15, *MUC5B* at 11p15, and *TERC* at 3q26, they also identified seven novel risk loci, such as *FAM13A* (4q22), *DSP* (6p24), *OBFC1* (10q24), *ATP11A* (13q34), *DPP9* (19p13), and chromosomal regions 7q22 and 15q14-15. These are the genes involved in host defence, cell-cell adhesion, and DNA repair and defects in these functions may be responsible for IIP development. On aggregate, these 10 genetic risk loci contributed to 31-33% of the variability in the risk of developing fibrotic IIP. Among the seven novel loci, *OBFC1* is associated with a short telomere length [28]. By conducting an imputation analysis using data from 1,616 cases and 4,683 controls, Fingerlin et al. [29] identified additional genetic risk variants in the human leukocyte antigen (HLA) region. They found two HLA alleles (e.g., DRB1*1501 and DQB1*0602) that were strongly associated with fibrotic IIPs and induced differential lung tissue HLA gene expression.

Noth et al. [27] performed a three-stage GWAS that involved an initial GWAS followed by two subsequent independent case-control studies in patients of European-American ancestry. A total of 1,410 IPF cases and 2,934 controls were included. The following SNPs were identified as risk variants for IPF susceptibility: *MUC5B* SNP (*rs35705950*) at 11p15.5, *TOLLIP* SNPs (*rs111521887, rs5743894, rs5743890*) at 11p15.59, and one *SPPL2C* SNP (*rs17690703*) at 17q21.31. Unlike the GWAS by Fingerlin et al. [26] Noth et al. [27] did not find any association with the *TERT* or *TERC* genes.

The novel variant *TOLLIP* rs5743890 SNP is a protective allele as it is associated with reduced susceptibility. If a patient develops IPF despite carrying the protective *TOLLIP rs5743890* allele, however, the mortality is increased by 65%. *TOLLIP* expression was decreased by up to 50% in individuals carrying the minor allele of rs5743894. Although both the *MUC5B* and *TOLLIP* genes reside in the same locus and are within 70 kilobases of each other [30], Noth et al. [27] used linkage disequilibrium data to show that the *MUC5B* and TOLLIP gene loci are separated by a recombination hotspot and are independent.

In 2017, Allen et al. [31] performed a GWAS with 2,760 patients with IPF and 8,561 controls from the United Kingdom (UK) in a two-stage analysis. Their analysis confirmed the previously known mutations, including mucin 5B (*rs35705950*) and desmoplakin (*DSP*) (*rs2076295*) and they also identified one novel mutation in the A-kinase anchoring protein 13 (*AKAP13*) (*rs62025270*). The minor allele of *rs35705950* was also associated with an increased lung tissue expression of *AKAP13*, which plays an important role in profibrotic signalling pathways. The main sites of *AKAP13* expression were in epithelial and lymphoid tissues.

In a recent publication, Moore et al. [32] studied the association between rare and common variants with IPF in a case-control study. They performed deep targeted resequencing of rare mutations (*TERT, TERC, RTEL1, PARN,*

TINF2, SFTPC, SFTPA2, and *ABCA3*) and the common variants in a large population of IPF cases (N=3,624) and controls (N=4,442). The *MUC5B* promoter variant *rs35705950* was the strongest common IPF risk variant with an odds ratio of 5.45 (95% CI: 4.91–6.06) for one copy of the risk allele and 18.68 (95% CI: 13.34–26.17) for two copies of the risk allele (p=9.60 x 10^{-295}).

The investigators also identified for the first time rare/uncommon variations in *FAM13A, MIR4457, CLPTM1L, RP13-870H17.3, MCF2L*, and *RNPS1* associated with IPF. The rare variants in *TERT, FAM13A, RTEL1, TOLLIP, SFTPC, SFTPA2, PARN,* and *TINF2* have proportionally small effects on the genetic risk of IPF at the population level, however. In a large genetic association study, Hobbs et al. [33] showed that *FAM13A* was shared by chronic obstructive pulmonary disease (COPD) and IPF, but that it has the opposite effect to the C allele at *rs2609260*, i.e., *FAM13A* has a protective effect in COPD.

4. FAMILIAL ILD

A statement on the evidence-based guidelines for diagnosis and treatment of IPF in 2011 defined familial interstitial pneumonia (FIP) as interstitial pneumonia affecting two or more members of the same primary biological family [5]. Van Moorsel et al. [34] used a more restrictive definition of FIP, however, defining it as two or more first-degree family members with IIP. In one of the first population-based studies of familial pulmonary fibrosis (FPF) in the UK, Marshall et al. [8] detected 57 cases of FPF in 21 families with an estimated 0.5–2.2% of IPF being familial (prevalence: 1.3 cases per million). Later studies have shown a higher frequency of 20% of IIP cases being FIP, however [35, 36]. Steele et al. [37] looked at a large series of FIP (111 families, 353 affected patients, and 360 unaffected patients) that showed an autosomal dominant mode of transmission with evidence of vertical transmission. They found that older age, male sex, and a history of cigarette smoking were important risk factors for the development of the disease within these families. Cigarette smoking had an independent effect on the development of FIP (odds ratio = 3.6; 95% CI: 1.3–9.8; p=0.01) and smoking as a risk factor in FIP is an example of gene-environment interactions in the development of pulmonary fibrosis. Another interesting feature in the cohort was phenotypic heterogeneity of IIP seen in 45% of the families. Histopathologically and radiologically, the most common pattern was usual interstitial pneumonia (UIP). The natural history of FIP is characterised by a period of asymptomatic lung involvement and subclinical interstitial abnormalities have been detected in 10-22% of non-affected FIP families [37]. Rosa et al. [38] similarly showed interstitial lung abnormalities in high-resolution chest tomography (HRCT) scans of the chest in 22% of asymptomatic relatives of FIP probands. The role of screening HRCT scans for family members of FPF patients is not clear, however. El-Chemaly et al. [39] reported a very slow progression of asymptomatic disease in FPF patients and the asymptomatic preclinical phase associated with heterozygous *TERT* mutation (R1084P) progressed to fibrotic lung disease over two to three decades. The asymptomatic *TERT* mutation carriers also show extrapulmonary manifestations and among the carriers, 40% presented with premature hair greying (before 30 years of age) vs. 5% in non-carriers [40]. A family history of pulmonary fibrosis is the strongest risk factor for IPF (odds ratio = 6.1, 95% CI: 2.3–15.9; p < 0.0001) [35]. Most FIP has an autosomal dominant inheritance pattern with reduced penetrance, indicating the presence of genetic rare variants that have a large effect [41]. Reduced penetrance means that the person has inherited the mutant genes but never develops the disease. The first-degree relatives of FIP patients are at particularly higher risk of developing ILD compared to the general population. For example, Kropski et al. [42] did extensive phenotyping of 75 asymptomatic first-degree relatives of FIP patients (mean age: 50.8 years.) using blood sampling, HRCT scanning, bronchoscopies with bronchoalveolar lavage (BAL), and transbronchial biopsies. The HRCT revealed interstitial changes in 11 out of 75 of the at-risk subjects (14%) and transbronchial biopsies detected abnormalities in 35.2% of the subjects. The at-risk subjects also demonstrated telomere shortening, endoplasmic reticulum (ER) stress, and an increased level of *MUC5B rs35705950* promoter polymorphisms. These molecular abnormalities in some subjects preceded abnormalities detected by HRCT scan or transbronchial lung biopsies. Adult patients with FPF have a clinical presentation similar to the sporadic variety of IPF, except for an earlier age of onset of 55 years compared to 68 years in the sporadic variety [8, 43]. Similarly, a retrospective study done at the Mayo Clinic did not find any differences in the clinical features or survival rates of patients with FIP and those with sporadic IPF [20].

5. SURFACTANT PROTEIN-RELATED GENES

Surfactant molecules maintain alveolar stability and pulmonary surfactant is a mixture of proteins and lipids that is synthesised, packaged, and secreted by alveolar type 2 cells (AT2) [44]. The site of synthesis is the ER of the AT2 cells and lipids constitute the major part of the molecules (90%), with proteins accounting for 10% of their weight. There are four types of surfactant proteins: (SP)-A1, SF-A2, SP-B, SP-C, and SP-D encoded by *SFTPA1*, A2, B, C, and D respectively. The surfactant proteins SP-B and SP-C are hydrophobic in nature and maintain alveolar stability by reducing the surface tension of the alveoli. The SP-A and SP-D are hydrophilic and contribute to innate immune defence [45]. Unlike SP-B, which is also secreted by Clara cells, SP-C is expressed exclusively in AT2 cells [46]. SF-C is synthesised as a 21-kD pro-SP-C in AT2 cells and undergoes proteolysis, which results in the secretion of the mature 3.7-kD protein via the lamellar bodies [47, 48]. The processing and secretion of SP-C is dependent on the ATP-binding cassette subfamily A member 3 (*ABCA3*), which is a lamellar body membrane protein expressed exclusively by AT2 cells [49, 50]. The gene for the SF-C protein is situated on the short arm of chromosome 8 (8p21) and is called the *SFTPC* gene [51]. The c-terminus of pro-SP-C contains a novel, highly conserved region of approximately 100 amino acids known as the BRICHOS domain. This domain has been identified in several previously unrelated proteins,e.g., BRI(2), which is related to familial British and Danish dementia (FBD and FDD); Chondromodulin-I (ChM-I), which is related to chondrosarcoma; and

CA11, which is related to stomach cancer [52]. The BRICHOS domain may play a role in the post-translational processing of surfactant proteins, including proper folding and trafficking [53].

5.1. *SFTPC* Mutations

The most frequently observed mutation in FPF is a mutation of the *SFTPC* gene [54] and the majority of mutations in the *SFTPC* gene occur in the C-terminal BRICHOS domain (exons 4 and 5) of the pro-SF-C protein [53]. Mutations in the BRICHOS region affect folding and conformational changes in the propeptide. In 2001, Nogee et al. [55] reported a mutation in the gene encoding SF-C in an infant and mother with FIP. The mother had desquamative interstitial pneumonitis (DIP), while the infant had cellular nonspecific interstitial pneumonitis (NSIP). The mutation involved was identified by a candidate-gene approach and included a heterozygous G to A transition at the first base of intron 4 (IVS4 +1G → A) of both patients, resulting in skipping of exon 4 with deletion of its 37 amino acids from the C-terminal domain of the immature pro-SP-C (SPCΔexon4). This mutation removes a consensus BRICHOS cysteine residue in the C-terminal region of the propeptide. By looking at the kindred of 11 individuals, Thomas et al. [56] identified an association between mutations in *SFTPC* and FIP. Six adults and three children had pathologic diagnoses of UIP and cellular NSIP, respectively. They identified a heterozygous missense +128T>A mutation in exon 5 of *SFTPC* that substituted glutamine for leucine at codon 188 of the propeptide (L188Q). This was the first report showing an association between *SFTPC* mutation and the pattern of UIP. The frequency of rare variants of the *SFTPC* gene in FPF is between 1% and 2% and *SFTPC* mutations have also been associated with adult familial IIP [57, 58]. In a study done with a Dutch cohort, Van Moorsel et al. [34] reported a 25% prevalence of *SFTPC* mutations among adult FPF patients and did not find any mutation in the sporadic cases. *SFTPC* mutation may also develop de novo. Brash et al. [59] reported a de novo heterozygous missense mutation of the *SFTPC* gene (g.1286T>C) in an infant with combined histological features of NSIP and PAP, resulting in a substitution of threonine for isoleucine at position 73 (I73T). The I73T is the most frequently found mutation in the human *SFTPC* gene [60, 61]. Mechri et al. [62] reported that patients with an *SFTPC* mutation had an I73T mutation in 50% of cases. Therefore, the genetic analysis should initially begin with a search for the I73T mutation before *SFTPC* gene sequencing [54]. Cottin et al. [63] reported for the first time the presence of a heterozygous mutation, I73T, in a mother with a diagnosis of combined pulmonary fibrosis and emphysema (CPFE) and her child. Pulmonary fibrosis caused by *SFTPC* mutations is a worldwide phenomenon as this has also been detected in an Asian cohort. In a Japanese cohort, Ono et al. [64] reported a novel heterozygous mutation, c.298G.A (G100S), in the BRICHOS domain of proSP-C, where the Glycine at codon 100 of *SFTPC* was mutated to serine. One interesting feature of the *SFTPC*^{G100S} mutation is the late onset and slow progression of respiratory symptoms, which is unlike other *SFTPC* mutations. Familial ILD with *SFTPC* mutations shows an autosomal dominant pattern of inheritance along with variable penetrance and phenotypic heterogeneity. The radiological pattern in adult familial patients is mainly the pattern of UIP, whereas in children, this includes NSIP, DIP, and pulmonary alveolar proteinosis (PAP). Sporadic cases of IPF also show *SFTPC* mutations, but at a lower frequency [65, 66]. Lawson et al. [65] evaluated the *SFTPC* mutations in 89 patients diagnosed with sporadic UIP and 46 patients with sporadic NSIP. They reported 10 SNPs in the *SFTPC* gene, but only one SNP produced a change in the amino acid sequence (I73T). The *SFTPC* mutation is characterised by highly variable age at onset and severity of lung disease, ranging from death in early infancy to development of pulmonary fibrosis in the fifth or sixth decade [56, 64]. It is inherited as autosomal dominant with incomplete penetrance, however, de-novo mutations may also occur. The *SFTPC* mutation may be related to the development of pulmonary fibrosis via several mechanisms. An in vitro study done by Wang et al. [67] showed that deletion of exon 4 from human *SFTPC* resulted in intracellular accumulation of incompletely processed and misfolded *SFTPC* proteins, known as aggresomes. These aggresomes produce a dominant-negative effect on the trafficking of co-expressed wild-type pro-SP-C protein. Nogee et al. [55] also showed that the levels of the transcripts encoding normal surfactant protein C precursor protein were similar to those of the transcripts encoding the abnormal protein. The BRICHOS domain mutations are associated with protein misfolding and aggresome formation in vitro. Ultimately, this causes apoptosis through multiple unfolded protein response (UPR) signalling pathways [53] and ER stress has also been reported in sporadic cases of IPF [68]. Non-BRICHOS domain mutations lead to fibrosis development through different mechanisms, however. In an in vitro study, Hawkins et al. [69] showed that a rare variant (Ile73Thr) within the non-BRICHOS domain led to impairment of protein autophagy and mitophagy, and subsequent epithelial cell dysfunction. This led to the alveolar epithelial cell becoming susceptible to 'second hits', which supports the current concept of the pathogenesis of IPF, i.e., the 'recurrent hit hypothesis' [70]. Similarly, Zhong et al. [71] demonstrated that ER stress in response to either chemical induction or overexpression of mutant *SFTPC* due to misfolding is associated with the epithelial-mesenchymal transition (EMT) in alveolar epithelial cells and can contribute directly to pulmonary fibrosis. ER stress may serve as a therapeutic target for the future [72].

5.2. *SFTPA2* Mutations

In a whole-genome linkage analysis of a large kindred with familial IPF and lung adenocarcinoma, Wang et al. [73] identified a susceptibility locus on chromosome 10q22 that contained the two genes *SFTPA1* and *SFTPA2*. They identified a missense mutation (GGG to GTG) in codon 231 of one *SFTPA2* allele, which contains a substitution of valine for a highly conserved glycine at codon 231 in *SFTPA2* (G231V). Wang et al. [73] reported another mutation in codon 198 (TTC to TCC), which substitutes serine for phenylalanine (F198S) in a second family. Both of these mutations are rare variants, as they were not detected in 3,557 multi-ethnic healthy controls. The segregation of adenocarcinoma lung with pulmonary fibrosis in the *SFTPA2* mutation carrier may explain the existence of a combined phenotype of both the diseases. Therefore, FPF co-segregating with lung cancer should alert the clinician to the need to search for *SFTPA2* mutations. Mutations in these two families are characterised by an early onset (<50 years) disease with autosomal dominant inheritance and high penetrance. Using a Dutch cohort of 39 FIP and 118 sporadic patients with IIP, Van Moorsel et al. [74] identified three new heterozygous mutations in exon 6 of *SFTPA2*: *N210T*, *G231R*, and *N171Y* genes. All these mutations, and those reported by Wang et al. [73] involved exon 6. Lung cancer was diagnosed in all *SFTPA2* families. The mechanism of pulmonary fibrosis in *SFTPA2* mutation is similar to that of patients with *SFTPC* mutations: protein misfolding and ER stress [73, 75]. The exact mechanism of tumorigenesis by ER stress is not known. In an experimental study, Zhu et al. [76] demonstrated that increased ER stress created a positive feed-forward loop by upregulating phosphorylated protein kinase B (p-AKT), which caused reduced senescence and the promotion of tumorigenesis. Additionally, Nathan et al. [77] showed a heterozygous missense mutation in *SFTPA1* (p.Trp211Arg) in families affected by IPF and lung adenocarcinoma. An interesting observation with *SFTPA1* mutation is the large variability in patient age that can be seen at the time of diagnosis, with patients ranging from infants to the elderly.

5.3. *ABCA3*

ATP-binding cassette 3 (*ABCA3*) transporters are transmembrane proteins that function by transporting macromolecules across biological membranes [78]. This process helps in alveolar surfactant secretion. *ABCA3*, belonging to subfamily A, member 3, is expressed exuberantly in AT2 cells and is localised on the lamellar bodies [79]. The *ABCA3* gene is located on chromosome 16 [44]. *ABCA3* mutations that cause lung diseases are inherited as an autosomal recessive pattern requiring mutations on both alleles; however, a compound heterozygous pattern has also been reported [80]. Shulenin et al. [81] in 2004, reported that *ABCA3* mutations were associated with severe, fatal respiratory distress in early infancy, with such infants requiring ventilatory support. The various mutations reported are homozygous nonsense, splice-site, missense, and frameshift mutations, as well as heterozygous insertion and splice-site mutations. Ultrastructural examination revealed abnormal lamellar bodies in AT2 cells. Studying a large Italian kindred, Campo et al. [82] diagnosed a novel homozygous G > A transition at nucleotide 2891, localised within exon 21, resulting in a glycine-to-aspartic acid change at codon 964 (*G964D*). This was associated with pulmonary fibrosis. Lung specimens taken from the young patient in the study showed features of the UIP pattern, whereas the two adult patients showed an NSIP pattern. *ABCA3* mutation was also reported in a 15-year-old boy, with a biopsy-proven UIP pattern and upper lobe–predominant radiographic findings [83]. The *ABCA3* mutation has been reported in a French patient, who showed combined pulmonary fibrosis and emphysema (CPFE) [84]. Sequence analysis revealed two mutations of the *ABCA3* gene: c.3081_3092delinsCG resulting in a serine to valine change at codon 1028 with the creation of a stop codon 103 amino acids downstream (p.Ser1028Valfs*103); and the common mutation c.875A.T, changing a glutamic acid to valine at codon 292 (p.Glu292Val). *ABCA3* mutations may modify the severity of lung disease in individuals with *SFTPC* mutation. Bullard et al. [85] reported *ABCA3* mutations in four severely affected infants with the same *SFTPC* mutation, a substitution of isoleucine by threonine in codon 73 (I73T). The heterozygous ABCA3 mutations were inherited from healthy parents without *SFTPC* I73T, clearly indicating that *ABCA3* acts as a modifier in the presence of an *SFTPC* mutation. The *ABCA3* mutation has also been detected in adult-onset fibrotic lung disease [86].

6. Genes Associated with Host Defence

6.1. Mucin 5B (*MUC5B*) Gene

Airway mucus is an important innate defence system of the lungs. The mucus barrier traps and eliminates inhaled particulates and pathogens daily via mucociliary clearance (MCC) [87, 88]. However, excessive mucus is also detrimental to human health, as it has been incriminated in the pathogenesis of numerous respiratory conditions [87]. The mucin genes *MUC5AC* and *MUC5B* are present as a conserved cluster on human chromosome 11p15; they encode the mucin glycoproteins in airway mucus, which causes the gel-like quality of the mucus [87, 89]. *MUC5B* is secreted from the bronchial glands; it is expressed in the cytoplasm of the goblet cells in the bronchi or the bronchioles (>200 µm) of the healthy lung. *MUC5B* is the dominant gel-forming mucin in a normal distal airway epithelium. Using a genome-wide linkage analysis of 82 patients with FIP, in 2011 Seibold et al. [90] reported an association between familial and sporadic pulmonary fibrosis and a 3.4-Mb region on chromosome 11p15. Subsequently, fine mapping using a case-control association analysis of 492 patients with IPF and 322 controls identified a SNP (*rs35705950*) in the putative *MUC5B* promoter region (3 kb upstream of the *MUC5B* transcription start site) that is significantly associated with the development of IPF and FPF. The major and minor alleles at the *rs35705950* SNP are guanine (G) and thymine (T), respectively. The T allele is most strongly associated with IPF. The minor allele of this SNP was detected in 38% of patients with sporadic IPF and 34% of patients with FIP, but only in 9% of controls (an overall allele frequency of 0.10). Allelic frequency in both sporadic and familial cases is very similar, indicating that the variant contributes substantially to both IPF and FIP. The allele frequency in the Caucasian control group in the study by Seibold et al. [90] is 9%, indicating that development of IPF occurs due to the interaction between gene and environment [91]. After controlling for *rs35705950*, the researchers reported only two other SNPs with nominal significance for IPF (*rs41480348*, p= 0.05; *rs12804004*, p = 0.02). The odds ratio for developing the disease for patients who are heterozygous (GT) and homozygous (TT) of the SNP (*rs35705950*) was 6.4 and 20.2 for FIP, and 9.0 and 21.8 for sporadic IPF, respectively. The *MUC5B* promoter variant *rs35705950* is the strongest risk factor, genetic or otherwise, for the development of pulmonary fibrosis [92]. The *MUC5B* polymorphism, *rs35705950*, contributes to 30% of the overall risk of IPF [26]. The significant association of the *rs35705950* SNP with IPF suggests a possible role played by the *MUC5B* gene in pulmonary fibrosis; this needs further evaluation. The SNP *rs35705950* is only associated with IPF, FIP and idiopathic non-specific interstitial pneumonia (NSIP) [93]; no association with sarcoidosis or systemic sclerosis-interstitial lung disease (SSc-ILD) has been reported. Stock et al. [94] evaluated the role played by the SNP (*rs35705950*) of the *MUC5B* gene in fibrotic lung disease, in the settings of SSc-ILD (n = 440) or sarcoidosis (n= 180) in a UK cohort. They reported a lack of association but noted instead that there was a significant association between the *MUC5B* SNP and IPF (odds ratio = 4.90, 95% CI: 3.42-7.03) in this cohort. A meta-analysis of the French, Italian and American cohorts conducted by Borie et al. [95] confirmed the lack of association between *MUC5B* SNP and SSc-ILD and a significant association with IPF. The odds ratios for IPF in heterozygous patients and homozygous patients are 6.3 [4.6–8.7] and 21.7 [10.4–45.3], respectively. This suggests that the *MUC5B* variant is specific to IPF-associated pulmonary fibrosis and that the fibrotic mechanism in scleroderma and sarcoidosis is different to that of IPF. The risk allele at *rs35705950* is a gain-of-function variant; as such, the expression of *MUC5B* is increased in the lung tissues from unaffected individuals and patients with IPF. IPF patients had a 14.1 times higher *MUC5B* expression in the lung compared to those who did not (P<0.001) regardless of genotype; however, the variant allele of *rs35705950* was associated with a 37.4-fold increase in *MUC5B* gene expression even in unaffected individuals [90]. Immunohistochemical staining shows *MUC5B* accumulation in the metaplastic epithelia lining the honeycomb cysts [90], terminal bronchiolar epithelial cells and in atypically differentiated cells in the bronchiolised distal airspaces of the IPF lung [96]. SSc-ILD is mainly associated with a NSIP that shows less architectural distortion, unlike the pattern seen in IPF patients.

The role of the rs35705950 variant in the pathogenesis of pulmonary fibrosis was further evaluated by Hunninghake et al. [97] in a population-based study that examined the Framingham Heart Study population. They reported an association between interstitial lung abnormalities seen in chest CTs and the *rs35705950* allele, determining a *rs35705950* minor allele frequency of 10.5%. After adjusting the covariates, Hunninghake et al. [97] established that one copy of the *rs35705950* allele increases the risk of radiographic interstitial lung abnormalities by 2.8 times and the risk of definite CT evidence of pulmonary fibrosis by 6.3 times. The interstitial lung abnormality seen on chest CTs may progress to overt ILD over time. This data suggests that genetic information may have the potential to allow an early diagnosis in asymptomatic patients. An increased number of copies of *MUC5B* promoter polymorphism and increasing age were associated with the long-term progression of interstitial lung abnormalities [98]. The association of polymorphism in the promoter region of *MUC5B* varies widely depending on the patient's race or ethnicity. The *MUC5B* promoter polymorphism SNP *rs35705950* is also a risk factor for IPF in the Mexican cohort (odds ratio= 7.36, P =0.0001), but not in the Korean cohort. (P=0.99). The allele frequency in the Korean cohort was 1%; it was absent in the Korean healthy controls [99]. Horimasu et al. [93] evaluated the association between *MUC5B* promoter polymorphism and IPF in a Japanese population and compared it with the German cohort. The *rs35705950* T allele frequencies in Japanese patients with IPF and NSIP, and those in the unaffected controls, were 3.4%, 1.7% and 0.8%, respectively; in comparison, they were 33.1%, 27.4%, and 4.3%, respectively among German patients. Wang et al. [100] reported the frequency of the T allele of *rs35705950* of 3.33% and 2.22% respectively in IPF and ILD patients in Chinese males, results which were significantly higher than those seen in the healthy controls (0.7%). Therefore, the *MUC5B* promoter mutation in Hispanic and Asian patients is shown to be considerably less frequent than in the Caucasian cohort. Interestingly, the promoter polymorphism of *MUC5B* indicated a survival advantage in patients with IPF. Peljto et al., using two large independent cohorts (INSPIRE and Chicago), found that *rs35705950* is significantly associated with better survival, independent of age, sex, pulmonary function, and treatment [101]. The exact reason for this survival benefit is not known. Stock et al. [94] also noted a trend towards a slower decline in forced vital capacity (FVC) among IPF patients with this polymorphism. Additionally, Cosgrove et al. [102] showed an association between the *MUC5B* promoter polymorphism and less-severe pathological changes in patients with FIP. Therefore, *MUC5B* polymorphism is unique in the sense that it not only promotes IPF development, but also reflects a significantly longer survival.

The exact reason for the IPF development due to polymorphism in the promoter region of the *MUC5B* gene is unknown, although several hypotheses have been put forward. IPF is considered a mucociliary disease and the *MUC5B* promoter variant *rs35705950* contributes to the overexpression of *MUC5B* in the distal airways of an IPF-affected lung [103, 104]. This leads to impaired mucociliary clearance, retention of inhaled particles, and lung injury. Ultimately, if prolonged, IPF may lead to fibrosis. After an injury to the bronchoalveolar regions of the lung, stem cells try to regenerate the injured bronchiolar and alveolar epithelia. However, an excess amount of *MUC5B* in the distal airways of IPF patients disrupts the normal regenerative process and may lead to aberrant repair, resulting in chronic fibroproliferation and honeycomb cyst formation [103]. The large size and extensively glycosylated *MUC5B* protein may be responsible for the failure of differentiation in stem cells. Honeycomb cyst development is more likely to occur due to an unsuccessful reparative process [103]. Yang et al. [105] demonstrated different molecular phenotypes of IPF based on gene expression profiles. Patients with a high expression of the cilium gene reveal more extensive microscopic honeycombing. They also showed an elevated lung tissue expression of *MUC5B* and *MMP7*, with the latter one implicated in attenuating ciliated cell differentiation during the wound repair process [106]. Lastly, large-sized and highly glycosylated *MUC5B* proteins lead to unfolded protein response and ER stress, which may interfere with the normal epithelial response to injury, wound healing, and tissue repair [107]. Chung et al. [108] demonstrated the effect of the *MUC5B* promoter polymorphism (*rs35705950*) on the CT imaging appearance of pulmonary fibrosis. The CT manifestation varies based on the underlying genotype. The T allele showed a greater proportion of confident UIP diagnoses (43.8% compared to 32.6% for the G group), whereas the G allele is more likely to show a CT imaging pattern that is inconsistent with UIP. No significant difference between the G and T groups regarding the presence of honeycombing was noted.

6.2. Toll-Interacting Protein (*TOLLIP*) Gene

TOLLIP is an ubiquitin-binding protein; it is an important regulator of innate immune defences mediated by the Toll-like receptor (TLR) and the transforming growth factor β (TGF-β) signalling pathway [109, 110]. The GWAS conducted by Noth et al. [27] identified an association between three *TOLLIP* SNPs (*rs111521887*, *rs5743894*, *rs5743890*) located in the genetic loci 11p15.5 and IPF susceptibility in European Americans. The susceptibility of SNP *rs5743890* also signifies IPF mortality. Fingerlin et al. [26] also identified *TOLLIP* SNPs in their GWAS but, after adjusting for the effect of *MUC5B* promoter SNP *rs35705950*, the effect of *TOLLIP* SNPs disappeared. This suggests that the linkage disequilibrium (LD) between *rs35705950* and *TOLLIP* is weak. The genetic loci for *TOLLIP* and *MUC5B* are same; that is, 11p15.5 and both genes are separated by 12 kb. (http://www.ncbi.nlm.nih.gov/gene/). However, the *TOLLIP* gene linked to IPF susceptibility is independent of the *MUC5B* promoter SNP.

Noth et al. [27] indicated a low LD between *MUC5B* and *TOLLIP* alleles. LD between the *MUC5B* promoter SNP (rs35705950) and *TOLLIP* SNPs (*rs111521887* [$r2=0.07$], *rs5743894* [$r2=0.16$], and *rs5743890* [$r2=0.01$]) was low, indicating that *TOLLIP* SNPs are independent of the *MUC5B SNPs*. Interestingly; the minor allele rs5743890 is a protective allele that lowers the risk of IPF. However; if an individual develops IPF despite the presence of the protective allele, this increases mortality [27]. Surprisingly, the *MUC5B* mutation at the same genetic locus had a survival benefit, indicating an independent association between *TOLLIP* and *MUC5B*. Oldham et al. [111] evaluated the relationship between SNP in *TOLLIP* and the response to *N*-acetylcysteine (NAC) therapy in IPF patients. Previously, the PANTHER trial had shown that NAC therapy is not helpful in IPF patients [112]. Oldham et al. [111] reported that NAC therapy was efficacious in IPF patients carrying the rs3750920 TT genotype, as it significantly reduced the composite endpoint risk (which includes death, hospitalisation, and FVC decline). However, those with the CC genotype showed a trend towards harm if treated with NAC. The TT genotype is present in 25% of IPF patients, suggesting that an important role will be played by pharmacogenetics in the future. *TOLLIP* is an inhibitory adaptor protein that inhibits TLR-mediated cytokine signalling. It also increases anti-inflammatory IL-10 production. TLR4 signalling can cause oxidant-dependent lung injury. The *rs3750920* polymorphism leads to uncontrolled TLR-mediated inflammation. NAC inhibits TLR-mediated inflammation and also increases the production of IL-10 [113]. However, why NAC therapy is useful only to the TT genotype is not known. O'Dwyer et al. [114] demonstrated *TLR3 L412F* polymorphisms which was associated with early mortality and accelerated lung function decline in IPF.

6.3. *ELMOD2*

Hodgson et al. [115] evaluated six multiplex families with FPF who originated from south-eastern Finland through a genome-wide scan. Further hierarchical fine mapping identified the engulfment and motility domain containing 2 (*ELMOD2*) gene as a novel candidate gene in FPF patients. The expression of the *ELMOD2* gene in the lung was significantly decreased in FPF patients. Indeed, 30% of affected family members and 7.7% of the Finnish controls shared a haplotype embodying *ELMOD2* and spanning 110 kb to 13 Mb on chromosome 4q31.1. The *ELMOD2* gene belongs to the group of six human proteins that take part in cellular processes such as the phagocytosis of apoptotic cells and cell migration [116, 117, 118]. The gene is expressed in lung epithelial cells and alveolar macrophages. Pulkkinen et al. demonstrated that the major downstream pathways of *ELMOD2* are involved in antiviral responses via the TLR3-mediated induction of type I and type III interferons [119]. In viral infection, *ELMOD2* expression is reduced; this supports the hypothesis that viral-induced epithelial injury is a trigger for IPF development.

6.4. Human Leukocyte Antigen (HLA)

The major histocompatibility complex (MHC) is located on the short arm of chromosome 6 (6p21.31) and contains the most polymorphic human leukocyte antigens (HLA) class I and II [120]. HLA functions mainly as a regulator of the immune response; certain HLA polymorphisms have shown a higher susceptibility to IPF [121, 122, 123]. The role of HLA in IPF susceptibility was demonstrated quite a while ago, when HLA typing was based on serology [124, 125, 126]. These days, with the advancement of molecular biology techniques, HLA typing has become more accurate and practical. Xu et al. [123] reported a significantly higher prevalence of DRB1*1501 among IPF patients than among controls. IPF patients carrying the DRB1*1501 allele had a 12% mean decrease in diffusing capacities for carbon monoxide (DLCO) compared to IPF patients without this allele. Falfan-Valencia et al. [121] showed that IPF patients carrying the DRB1*04 alleles had a significantly reduced epithelial growth rate, epithelial cell apoptosis and DNA breaks on BAL fluid analysis. Epithelial cell apoptosis is an important step in the development of IPF. Zhang et al. [122] reported a gene frequency of 10% with HLA-B*15, while Varpela et al. [126] similarly showed a potential association of HLA-B*15 with IPF pathogenesis. Fingerlin et al. [29] performed a genome-wide imputation-based association analysis of non-Hispanic Whites with fibrotic idiopathic interstitial pneumonias (1,616 cases and 4,683 control subjects). They subsequently replicated their findings using an independent cohort (878 cases and 2,017 control subjects). In this later study, they identified one novel locus in the HLA region of chromosome 6p21. (rs7887 Pmeta = 3.7×10^{-09}) and two HLA alleles, DRB1*15:01 and DQB1*06:02, associated with fibrotic idiopathic interstitial pneumonias. Fingerlin et al. [29] also performed targeted RNA-sequencing of the HLA locus, identifying 21 genes differentially expressed between fibrotic and control lung tissue. Many of these genes play key roles in immune and inflammatory response regulation. These two alleles (DRB1*15:01 and DQB1*06:02) contribute to a 35% variability in the risk of developing fibrotic idiopathic interstitial pneumonias. The HLA associations may suggest that autoimmunity plays a role in the pathogenesis of ILD. Falfan-Valencia et al. [127] assessed the role of MHC in disease susceptibility through a study of 19 related Mexican patients with hypersensitivity pneumonitis (HP), 25 healthy first-degree relatives and 246 healthy unrelated individuals. Using molecular genotyping and polymerase chain reaction (PCR), Falfan-Valencia et al. [127] identified a significantly increased frequency in the following HLA alleles in individuals with HP compared to controls: HLA-DRB1*04:07, DRB1*04:05, DRB1*11:01 and DRB1*13:01 (P value<0.05). They also detected the TNF-238 GG genotype more frequently in the HP group, compared with its frequency in the control subjects. The DRB1*15 and DQB1*06 alleles have been associated with interstitial lung disease in a sample of rheumatoid arthritis patients in Japan, whereas the HLA-DRB1 shared epitopes were associated with a reduced risk of ILD [128]. Aquino-Galvez et al. [129] found a significantly increased level of the MHC class I chain-related gene A (MICA) MICA*001 in IPF patients (OR = 2.91). The MICA expression was localised to alveolar epithelial cells and fibroblasts from IPF lungs, but it was not found in control lungs.

The expression of the MICA receptor NKG2D was also significantly reduced in natural killer cells (NK cells) and gamma-delta T cells from IPF lungs. MICA, by interacting with NKG2D receptors, provides a costimulatory signal for the activation of NK cells, resulting in the lysis of altered epithelial cells. MICA polymorphisms fail to remove the altered alveolar epithelial cells. The aberrantly activated alveolar epithelial cells not only produce pro-fibrotic mediators but also undergo an epithelial–mesenchymal transition if they escape lysis [130, 131]. There are two mechanisms by which MICA polymorphisms fail to remove altered alveolar epithelial cells: first, polymorphisms reduce MICA binding to NKG2D receptors; second, the soluble form of MICA (once released) down-regulates the activity of NKG2D by promoting its internalisation and degradation [132]. Table-1 shows various HLA that are linked to ILD.

Table 1. Is Showing HLA Linked to ILD

Evans C. 1976.(133)	HLA B12
Strimlan et al. 1977 (134)	No significant associations with any antigen; however, HLA-B15 was non-significantly increased in the patient group.
Turton et al. 1978. UK (125)	HLAB8 The association was highest in patients with onset of disease before the age of fifty and women
Varpela et al. 1979. Finland. (126)	**HLA-B15** and HLA-Dw6
Falfan-Valencia et al. 2005 Mexico (127)	DRB1*01 (OR=10.72) DRB1*14 (OR=4.42) DRB1*04 (OR=4.73).
Aquino-Galvez et al. 2009. Mexico (129)	MHC class I chain-related gene A (MICA) MICA*001 was significantly increased in IPF patients (OR = 2.91).
Xu et al. 2011. USA (123)	DRB1*1501 Prevalent in IPF vs. Controls (33.1% vs. 20.0%, respectively, OR 2.0; 95%CI 1.3–2.9, p = 0.0004). Decreased in DLco among IPF patients with DRB1*1501
Zhang et al. 2012, Han Chinese population (122)	HLA-A*3, HLA-B*14, HLA-B*15, HLA-B*40
Zhang et al. 2015 China (135)	HLA-A*02-DRB1*04 (OR = 4.69)
Fingerlin et al. 2016 non-Hispanic White (NHW) cases (29)	DRB1*15:01 and DQB1*06:02

7. GENES ASSOCIATION WITH INFLAMMATION

7.1. Interleukin-1 (IL-1)

IL-1 is a cytokine with proinflammatory and fibrogenic effects. Members of the IL-1 gene family include IL-1α, IL-1β, and the IL-1 receptor antagonist (IL-1Ra) [136]. The genes encoding IL-1α, IL-1β, and IL-1Ra are clustered on chromosome 2q13–21 [137]. Whyte et al. [138] demonstrated that the +2018C>T allele of IL-1 Ra (SNP rs419598) and the *TNF-α* allele -308G>A have been associated with IPF in the British and Italian populations. Barlo et al. [139] showed that the G allele of rs2637988 SNP in the*IL1RN gene* was associated with a risk of IPF and a reduced level of BAL fluid IL-1Ra/IL-1β ratios. In a meta-analysis of five case-control studies conducted on the Caucasian population, Korthagen et al. [140] showed that polymorphisms in the variable number tandem repeat in the IL-1Ra gene (IL-1RN)(rs408392 and rs419598), increasing the subject's susceptibility to IPF. The IL1RN risk allele is associated with lower levels of IL-1Ra and predisposes individuals to fibrogenesis.

7.2. Transforming Growth Factor- β (*TGF-β*)

TGF-β is a key fibrogenic cytokine that has been implicated in pulmonary fibrosis. It produces fibrosis by multiple mechanisms such as fibroblasts recruitment, enhanced proliferation, and differentiation of fibroblasts, collagen production, enhanced EMT and inhibition of collagen degradation [141]. The *TGF-β$_1$* gene polymorphism T869C confers risk to IPF susceptibility among Koreans [142]. The TT genotype was also significantly associated with decreased PaO$_2$ and increased D(A–a)O$_2$ upon initial diagnosis (p = 0.006 and 0.009, respectively), thereby indicating disease severity. The *TGF-β$_1$* gene is located on chromosome 10q13. Xaubet et al. [143] found that *TGF-β1* polymorphisms in codons 10 and 25 (+869 T>C and +915 G>C) do not increase the risk of IPF development. However, they demonstrated that the pro allele in codon 10 of *TGF-β1* gene was independently associated with worsening of gas exchange.

8. GENES ASSOCIATED WITH EXTRACELLULAR MATRIX

8.1. Matrix Metalloproteinases (*MMPs*)

MMPs play a key role in pulmonary fibrosis via regulation of extracellular matrix remodelling and several mediators such growth factors, cytokines, chemokines, and cell-surface-receptors [144]. Studies have shown that *MMP1* and *MMP7* are significantly overexpressed in IPF lungs compared to controls [145, 146]. In a case-control study conducted by Checa et al. [147] on 130 IPF patients and 305 healthy controls, the researchers found a higher frequency in the *MMP1* 2G polymorphism at position -1,607 (62 vs. 49%, p < 0.008; OR: 1.7, 95% CI: 1.15–2.79) in IPF patients compared to its frequency in controls. The investigators also studied the T/G SNP at position -755, finding no significant differences between IPF patients and healthy controls. However, when the study individuals were stratified according to their smoking status, the researchers noticed a significant increase in the T/T genotype frequency in smokers with IPF compared to its frequency in smoking controls (45 vs. 26%; P = 0.03; OR = 2.3; CI 1.15–4.97). This is an example of putative gene–environment interaction in patients with IPF.

9. GENES ASSOCIATED WITH CELL SENESCENCE

9.1. Telomere-Associated Gene Mutations

Telomeres are heterochromatic nucleoprotein structures consisting of the Hexamer 5'-TTAGGG-3' repeat that stabilize the chromosomal ends. Telomeres length is shortened successively with each cell division due to progressive loss of the TTAGGG repeat caused by the "end-replication" problem as well as degradation by nucleases enzymes [148]. The average rate of shortening with each cell division is 50 to 200 base pairs [149], and below a critical threshold (known as the Hayflick limit), short telomeres activate the p53-dependent checkpoint that results in cellular senescence and apoptosis [150]. Telomerase is an RNA-dependent DNA polymerase that synthesizes telomeric DNA by adding TTAGGG repeats onto the ends of chromosomes de novo [151]. Telomerase has two essential components: telomerase reverse transcriptase (*TERT*) and an RNA component (*TERC*). The *TERC* is a noncoding RNA that provides the template for the addition of six nucleotides telomeric repeats (*TTAGGG*) onto the 3' end of chromosomes by *TERT* [152]. In the adult, telomerase activity is confined to germ cells and stem cells [148]. Dyskerin is an accessory telomerase protein located on the X-chromosome *DKC1* gene and helps in biogenesis and stability of telomerase [152]. Dyskerin maintains *TERC* integrity by binding to an RNA motif within *TERC* known as the H/ACA domain [153, 154]. These components are important in order to maintain telomere length and genetic stability [155]. The *TERT* gene is located on the chromosome 5p15.33 (gene ID: 7015), whereas the *TERC* gene is on chromosome 3q26.2 (gene ID: 7012).

Tissues with high proliferative activity are susceptible to the detrimental effect of telomere length shortenings such as skin, bone marrow, and the bronchoalveolar epithelium. Heterozygous mutations of *TERT* or *TERC* genes had been reported initially in patients with dyskeratosis congenita (DKC) which is a rare hereditary disorder initially described by the triad of mucocutaneous manifestations such as skin hyperpigmentation, oral leukoplakia, and nail dystrophy. Bone marrow failure due to aplastic anaemia or complications of its treatment is the most common cause of death in patients with DKC, accounting for 67% of cases [10]. Pulmonary complication develops in approximately 20% of patients and is the second most common cause of death [10]. DKC is genetically heterogeneous and is transmitted by autosomal or X-linked inheritance pattern. The X-linked form is the most severe form which manifests in the first decade of life and is caused by mutation of the *DKC1* gene [157], whereas the autosomal dominant form has a later presentation, and is characterized by mutations in telomerase RNA (*TERC*) gene [158].

9.2. Rare Variant Mutations of Telomere-Related Genes

Genetic mutations of the telomerase gene are the most frequent genetic defect found in patients with autosomal dominant pulmonary fibrosis [158, 159]. The rare variants of the telomere-related gene mutations have been reported in both FIP and sporadic cases of IPF. Mutations in the *TERT* and *TERC* components of telomerase lead to shortened telomere length and development of pulmonary fibrosis. The rare variant mutations of telomerase genes show an autosomal dominant pattern of inheritance with variable penetrance. Families with telomere-related gene mutations also show anticipation with earlier and more severe manifestations in subsequent generations [160]. Accumulation of short telomeres in successive generations explains the phenomenon of anticipation and also highlights the fact that both a short telomere length and telomerase mutations determine disease onset and severity. Anticipation has been reported with mutations of the following rare variants in FPF patients: *TERT*, *TERC*, and *RTEL1* [57, 161, 162]. The phenotype of pulmonary fibrosis is age-dependent, as none of the *TERT* mutation carriers with age of less than 40 years develop pulmonary fibrosis, whereas 60% of men and 50% of women of age ≥ 60 years respectively have pulmonary fibrosis [159, 160]. The disease penetrance is much higher with telomere-related gene mutations than with mutations of the common variant, *MUC5B* gene. A substantial number of 40% harbouring the *TERT* mutation develop pulmonary fibrosis compared to <1% individuals carrying the *MUC5B* mutations who develop IPF [159]. Patients of telomere-related gene mutations also show considerable phenotypic heterogeneity as discordant diagnoses for individuals with an identical mutation can occur in up to 80% of families [161]. The frequency of *TERT* mutations is higher than *TERC* mutations, but the clinical features don't distinguish the mutant gene [163]. The heterozygous loss of function mutation of telomerase-related genes has been identified in up to 25% of FPF cases and 1-3% of sporadic cases of IPF respectively [164, 165, 166]. Among patients with telomere-related mutations and ILDs, IPF is the most frequent manifestation seen in approximately 65% of patients [24, 167]. Other ILDs associated with telomere-related mutations include NSIP, CHP, and cryptogenic organizing pneumonia. Therefore; telomere-related mutations increase the susceptibility to ILD in general, not to any specific types [163].

Armanios et al. [168] identified a three-generation kindred with features of autosomal dominant dyskeratosis congenita and a null *TERT* allele and the pedigree showed transmission of pulmonary fibrosis without skin manifestation and anticipation in successive generations. The mutation leads to haploinsufficiency of telomerase where the remaining functional copy of the gene failed to preserve normal telomerase function resulting in shortening of telomere in successive generations and development of anticipation. Armanios et al. [169] subsequently screened 73 probands with IPF from the Vanderbilt Familial Pulmonary Fibrosis Registry and identified six novel heterozygous germline mutations in *TERT* or *TERC in* 6 (8%) probands, all of which led to a decrease in telomerase activity. Five *TERT* mutations (2 missense, 2 slice junction, and one Frameshift) and one *TERC* mutations were detected. The mutated telomerase led to the development of short telomeres in peripheral blood lymphocytes, thereby even the asymptomatic mutant carriers are at risk of IPF. By using genome-wide linkage scan of chromosome 5p15 in two of the largest Caucasian families with familial IPF, Tsakiri et al. [165] identified two *TERT* mutations (Frameshift and missense mutation) that were cosegregated with pulmonary disease in the two families. By sequencing the probands of 44 unrelated families and 44 cases of sporadic IPF, the investigators identified five additional *TERT* mutations and one *TERC* mutation. The mutations were heterozygous meaning that a 50% reduction in enzyme activity was sufficient for disease initiation. However, the disease penetrance is variable as some family members showed features of DKC such as osteoporosis/osteopenia, anaemia and cancer but lacked the classical mucocutaneous manifestations. Individuals who were carrying the heterozygous mutations had a significantly shorter telomere length compared with normal family members, thereby increasing the susceptibility to adult-onset IPF. Unlike *SFTPC* mutations, patients with telomere-related mutations develop the pulmonary disease during adult life without any preceding history of paediatric lung disease. IPF is an example of adult-onset presentations of a Mendelian disorder as the mean age of patients with IPF and telomerase mutations is 51 years [159, 170].

9.3. Short Telomeres Length

Shortened telomere length is a risk factor for IPF development. Patients with telomerase mutation usually manifest with shortening of telomere in peripheral blood mononuclear cells (PBMC) and alveolar epithelial cells

[40, 163]. However, telomere length shortening has been identified in both familial and sporadic IPF patients, even in the absence of telomerase gene mutations. Cronkhite et al. [163] reported that 20-25% of patients with familial or sporadic IPF had telomere lengths less than the 10th percentile but did not have any detectable mutations. One reason may be due to the fact that not all mutations have been detected. Telomere length must be compared with age-adjusted controls as there is an age-related decline in telomere length in a normal person from 20 to 80 years by 20% [163]. Cronkhite et al. reported a short telomere length in 24% probands with FPF and 23% of sporadic pulmonary fibrosis cases without any detectable coding mutation of *TERT* or *TERC* genes [163]. IPF was the most common underlying diagnosis seen in 50-85% of patients with idiopathic interstitial pneumonia. Approximately, 15% of patients with mutations in *TERT* or *TERC* genes had telomere length above the 10th percentile. Development of pulmonary fibrosis is an age-related phenomenon as all patients with a heterozygous mutation in *TERT* or *TERC* with pulmonary fibrosis are more than 48 years of age and had short telomere. Diaz de Leon et al. [159] demonstrated similarly that the phenotype of pulmonary fibrosis is an age-dependent phenomenon. The investigators characterized 134 heterozygous *TERT* mutation carriers from 21 unrelated families with age ranging from 5 to 88 years, including 53 individuals with pulmonary fibrosis. Development of pulmonary fibrosis in *TERT* mutation carriers was age-dependent and associated with environmental exposures such as smoking. None of the patients with *TERT* mutations and age less than 40 years had pulmonary fibrosis but 60% and 50% of men and women of age ≥ 60 years, respectively, have pulmonary fibrosis. The mean age of men with *TERT* mutation was 54 years, younger than women patients with *TERT* mutation or patients with sporadic IPF. A history of exposure to smoking and/or a fibrogenic environmental or occupational agent has been reported in over 95% of *TERT* mutation carriers and a significant association between smoking and/or fibrogenic exposures with pulmonary fibrosis in *TERT* mutation carriers who are ≥40 years of age has been reported. Majority of patients (74%) had a UIP pattern on HRCT scan.

The mean survival of patients with *TERT* mutation-associated pulmonary fibrosis is 3 years after diagnosis; therefore, it is equally lethal similar to sporadic IPF. Diaz de Leon et al. [159] also studied the relationship between environmental exposure and IPF penetrance in patients *TERT* mutation carriers and age ≥40 years and reported the following odds ratio; personal history of smoking [OR 4.0 (1.2-14.5), P-value= 0.02] and/or other fibrogenic exposures [OR 13.6 (1.7-636.8), P-value=0.005]. Codd et al. [28] identified five loci containing candidate genes (*TERC, TERT, NAF1, OBFC1,* and *RTEL1*) that are known to be involved in telomere biology along with lead SNPs at two loci (*TERC* and *TERT*) associated with several cancers and other diseases, including IPF.

Alder et al. reported a significantly short telomeres length than the age-matched controls [166]. The shortening occurs not only in peripheral blood lymphocytes and granulocytes but also involves the alveolar epithelial cells. About 3% of sporadic IPF patients with a short telomere had cryptogenic liver cirrhosis suggesting the role of short telomeres in extrapulmonary organ involvement. These cohorts lack apparent telomerase mutations. Patients with *TERC* diseases-associated variants have the shortest telomere length, suggesting an increased penetrance and higher risk or telomere syndrome in this group [166]. Telomere length is a heritable trait. Parents with *TERT* mutation transmit the short telomeres to offspring which shortens in successive generations. The non-mutational carriers may also have short telomeres due to ancestral effect [171]. Alder et al. [172] identified six non-mutational carrier individuals with short telomere. One patient with short telomere also had clinical evidence of ILD. Therefore, parental telomere length may be contributed to telomere shortening and risk of ILD in the patient. Short telomere length is also a poor prognostic marker. Snetselaar et al. [173] had shown that the shortest telomere length was found in alveolar type 2 (AT2) cells within the fibrotic areas and indicates a shorter survival. The length of telomere was 56% longer in the non-fibrotic areas compared to fibrotic areas in sporadic IPF patients. Apart from AT2 cells, no difference in telomere length was found in surrounding cells, suggesting a possible role of AT2 cells in fibrogenesis. Planas-cerezales et al. [174] in a study done in Spanish and Mexican cohort showed that sporadic IPF patients with age less than 60 years and/or presenting with non-specific immunological or haematological abnormalities had a high predictive risk of telomere shortening. The outcome was also poor in younger patients.

9.4. Extrapulmonary Manifestations of Telomerase-Related Mutation

Mutations in *TERT/TERC* are also associated with extra-pulmonary abnormalities involving skin, liver and haematological abnormalities and this entity is called telomere syndrome. Following features should be noted in patients with ILD, particularly with a family history; abnormal blood count, liver abnormalities such as repeated unexplained elevated liver enzyme levels or liver disease and cutaneous abnormalities (hair greying before the age of 30, skin hyperpigmentation, oral leukoplakia, and nail dystrophy). One prevailing concept is that the different diseases related to telomere dysfunction are seen in different individuals of the same family rather than the same individual. However, affected individuals often manifest involvement of other organs subclinically, even when symptoms related to a single disorder predominate [160, 168]. George et al. [175] reported subclinical organ involvement among 13 patients with ILD and short telomeres referred for lung transplantation. About 53% of patients had bone marrow abnormalities, most commonly hypocellular marrow with macrocytosis and relatively normal counts. Phenotypic manifestation depends on the generation involved. Mutations in older generations manifest clinically as adult-onset pulmonary fibrosis, whereas, mutations in later generations more frequently present in childhood with aplastic anaemia along with classic features of DC. Patients with IPF who have mutant telomerase genes are at an increased risk of developing bone marrow failure and liver disease. In the Alder et al. [166] series, four patients (3%) had a history of unexplained liver cirrhosis out of 150 IIP patients. All these patients had short telomere without having any detectable telomerase mutations. Few patients in this cohort probably had subclinical aplastic anaemia. Parry et al. [170] had reported co-occurrence of aplastic anaemia and pulmonary fibrosis in a single individual, suggestive of a germline telomere maintenance defect. Detection of concurrent bone marrow involvement is important as it determines the choice of immunosuppressive drugs in patients undergoing transplantation. Diaz de Leon et al. [159] reported anaemia in 13.4% cases and aplastic anaemia in 3.0% cases, elevated liver function test in 8.2% of cases of *TERT* mutation carriers and one *TERT* mutation carrier had cryptogenic liver cirrhosis. Macrocytosis, graying of hair has also been reported [40, 176]. Telomerase-related mutations are loss-of-function mutations manifest as an autosomal dominant pattern of inheritance with the feature of anticipation. Anticipation is characterized by an early onset and more severe phenotypes occurring in successive generations [162, 168]. This occurs due to the accumulation of short telomeres in successive generations.

9.5. Other Telomerase-Gene Related Mutations

TERT or *TERC* mutations have not been detected in many patients of FPF and sporadic IPF with shortened telomere length. Other genes involved in telomere maintenance may explain length shortening. *RTEL1*, *PARN*, *DKC1*, and *TINF2* are other less common variants of telomerase-related genes that have been identified in patients with pulmonary fibrosis. Stuart et al. [177] performed whole-exome sequencing (WES) of genomic DNA samples from 99 probands with familial pulmonary fibrosis of unknown genetic cause and identified two gene variants in 78 European cases of ILD in comparison with 2,816 European controls. They found an exoribonuclease, *PARN* with five new heterozygous mutations shared by all affected relatives (odds in favor of linkage = 4,096:1). They also reported damaging and missence mutations in *RTEL1* gene at a significantly greater frequency than controls. Both mutation carriers were associated with shortened telomere length. The *PARN* and *RTEL1* gene mutations are responsible for 7% of familial pulmonary fibrosis patients. The regulator of telomere elongation helicase 1 (*RTEL1*) is a DNA helicase enzyme that helps in telomere replication and stability. DNA helicase helps in the unwinding of the T-loop structure at telomeric ends [178]. *RTEL1* deficiency results in progressive telomere shortening as the endonuclease SLX4 enzyme causes cleavage of the telomeric ends proximal to the T-loop, releasing the circular fragments of telomeric DNA as T-circle [179]. *RTEL1* is located on chromosome 20q13.33. In another WES-based study of FPF patients, Cogan et al. identified a rare heterozygous loss-of-function mutation of *RTEL1* gene in 4.7% of the kindreds which segregated with clinical FIP. It was associated with severe telomere length shortening (<10th percentile for age) in the peripheral blood mononuclear cells (PBMC) and increased T-circle formation [180]. Mutations in *TERT*, *TERC*, *DKC1*, and *RTEL1* contribute to one-third of FIP patients with short telomere.

Kannengiesser et al. had reported a higher frequency of heterozygous *RTEL1* mutations (11%) among 35 families with FPF [181]. Similar to *TERT* mutation carriers, patients of FPF with *RTEL1* mutations also show the phenomenon of anticipation. Exposure to smoking and other fibrogenic stimuli were also higher, indicating the role of gene-environment interaction in disease development. Penetrance may also depend on environmental factors [159]. In patients with *RTEL1* mutations, alkylating agents should be used with caution [181]. Through its role in genomic stability and replication, *RTEL1* may confer additional risk. Inherited mutations in *RTEL1* gene have been reported in Hoyeraal-Hreidarsson syndrome, characterized by accelerated telomere shortening, immunodeficiency, and developmental defects [182]. Borie et al. [183] evaluated the phenotype of patients with ILD and carriers of *RTEL1* heterozygous mutation. *RTEL1* mutation carrier was identified by whole exome sequencing and a total of 35 patients from 17 independent families with ILD and a pathogenic *RTEL1* mutation was identified. The ILD diagnosis included IPF (n=20, 57%) secondary ILD (n=7, 20%) and unclassifiable fibrosis or IPAF (n=7, 20%). Median age at diagnosis was 55.2 years. IPF was the most common diagnosis, found in 57& of patients. Other alternative diagnosis included IPAF (17.2%), RA-ILD (11.4%), chronic HP (5.7%), sarcoidosis and pneumoconiosis (one patient each). Compared to other telomere-related gene mutations, extra-pulmonary manifestations are less common. Hematological abnormalities and hepatic disease were found in 22% and

11% of patients of ILD with *RTEL1* mutations respectively. The corresponding values in *TERT* were 61% and 36% respectively, whereas, in *TERC* mutations, it is 50% each. The investigators also reported a mean FVC decline of 140.5 mL/year.

Dressen et al. [184] in a whole-genome sequencing study included 1510 patients with IPF and 1874 non-IPF controls assessed telomere length and compared enrichment of rare protein-altering variants, stratified by rs35705950 genotype. A rare variant was defined by a minor allele frequency (MAF) of less than 1%. The investigators reported a significant enrichment of rare variants in *TERT* gene among patients who did not carry any copies of the *MUC5B* risk allele as 34 (7%) of 464 individuals who did not carry a risk allele at *MUC5B* had rare functional variants in *TERT* compared with 30 (3%) of 1046 *MUC5B* risk allele carriers. (odds ratio 0·40 [95% CI 0·24–0·66], p=0·00039). Dressen et al. [184] also assessed the rate of disease progression based on the mean percentage decrease in predicted FVC in patients from the placebo arms of the ASCEND and CAPACITY clinical trials and demonstrated a more rapid decline in predicted FVC in patients with a rare variant of *TERT*, *PARN*, *TERC*, or *RTEL1* than patients without a single variant (1.66% vs 0.83% per month, P=0.02). On the contrary, IPF patients with the *MUC5B* risk allele were older than patients without the risk allele (mean age 68.1 years [SD 7.6] *vs* 65.5 years [8.3]; p<0.0001) and had a slower disease progression. The mean telomere length in IPF patients with rare variants *TERT*, *PARN*, *TERC*, and *RTEL1* were 2.93 (0.66), 2.57 kb (SD 0.62), 2.32 kb (0.68), and 2.57 kb (0.52) respectively with a mean telomere length shorter by 348 bp per variant than patients without the variant. This study defines two subsets of patients genetically; IPF with telomere-related mutation and IPF with *MUC5B* mutations. The exact mechanism by which *RTEL1* is associated with pulmonary fibrosis is unknown, however; Borie et al. [183] demonstrated localization of *RTEL1* in epithelial cells and not in fibroblastic foci. Therefore, it is possible that *RTEL1* is associated with alveolar epithelial dysfunction.

Alder et al. [185] by exome sequencing identified mutations in the telomere binding protein, *TINF2* in patients with FPF. *TINF2* mutation is a rare cause of pulmonary fibrosis responsible for 1% of mutations seen in patients with FPF. They identified the following mutations; a 15-base-pair deletion encompassing the exon 6 splice acceptor site, and a missense mutation, Thr284Arg. The deletion was an acquired phenomenon and may show a protective advantage by diminishing the expression of the missense mutation. The *TINF2* mutation has also been linked to infertility which preceded the onset of pulmonary fibrosis. Testing for telomere-related mutations should be considered in the presence of a family history of infertility in patients with pulmonary fibrosis. Besides *TINF2* mutations, male and female infertility preceding pulmonary fibrosis has been reported in 11% of *TERT* and *TERC* mutation carriers [185]. *TINF2* is one of the components of the shelterin complex, which facilitates the recruitment of telomerase to telomeres [186]. *TINF2* mediates this action via both TPP1-dependent and independent pathway. Among various genes implicated in DC, mutations in *TERC, TERT*, and *DKC1* have been found to be associated with FPF and IPF. *TINF2* mutation has also been identified in DC patients with pulmonary fibrosis [187]. Petrovski et al. [188] by exome sequencing methods identified that 11.3% of sporadic IPF also carried mutations in one of the three genes; *TERT, RTEL1*, and *PARN*, indicating genetic commonalities between the FPF and sporadic variety. The *PARN* gene is responsible for the biogenesis of *TERC* [189]. The genetic model in ILD is probably oligogenic as the *MUC5B* promoter risk allele (rs35705950 [G>T] is significantly elevated among patients with mutations of *TERT, RTEL1* and *PARN* variants [188].

There are no interactions among various mutations. Previous studies related to genetics in IPF have focussed mainly on a single gene. Coghlan et al. [190] studied the frequency and interactions of six IPF-related genes, including *SFTPA2, SFTPC*, ABCA3, *TERT*, thyroid transcription factor (*NKX2-1*) and *MUC5B* in 132 patients with IPF and compared it with 192 individuals with chronic obstructive pulmonary disease (COPD) and the population represented in the Exome Variant Server. The IPF cohorts consisted of both sporadic and familial variety. The investigators observed 15 mutations in 14 individuals in the IPF cohort: *SFTPA2, SFTPC, TERT*, and *ABCA3*. No individual with IPF had two different mutations, indicating a lack of interactions among these genes. Presence of mutations linked to childhood ILD in an adult with IPF indicates that these mutations can contribute to a spectrum of ILDs manifesting at all ages.

9.6. Prognosis

Telomerase mutations portend a poor prognosis in IPF patients. Pulmonary fibrosis associated with *TERT* mutation is progressive and lethal with a mean survival of 3 years after diagnosis [159]. Newton et al. [161] had shown that ILD associated with mutations in telomere-related genes had a uniformly progressive disease with the mean rate of FVC decline of 300 ml/year compared to 130-210 ml/year reported in the placebo arm of multiple IPF clinical trials [191]. The median time to death or transplant was 2.87 years. However; no significant difference in the time to death or transplant for different gene mutations or for patients with a clinical diagnosis of IPF or non-IPF ILD was reported, thereby obviating the need for a surgical lung biopsy. Newton et al. [161] had shown certain salient differences in clinical manifestations depending on underlying mutations. Patients with *TERC* mutations had a more frequent occurrence of severe haematological diseases, whereas radiographic emphysema was significantly associated with *TERT* and *RTEL1* gene mutations. Subjects with *RTEL1* mutations also showed a significantly higher frequency of lung cancer compared to other groups. Shorter telomere length is a poor prognostic marker in patients with IPF. The telomere length has been recorded in the following order in telomere gene mutations from shortest to longest; *TERC<TERT<RTEL1<PARN*. The mean age of onset of ILD is related to the degree of telomere shortening and follows the same pattern with an earlier occurrence in *TERC* mutation carriers (51 years) compared to mutation carriers of *TERT* (58 years), *RTEL1* (60 years) and *PARN* (64 years) genes.

The outcome of lung transplantation in IPF patients with underlying telomerase mutations showed poor results in retrospective case series [192, 193, 194]. One retrospective cohort of 9 patients from France showed that patients with telomerase mutations had an increased the risk of severe hematologic complications, in particular, bone marrow failure after lung transplantation with a post-transplant median survival of 214 days [192]. Therefore; proper risk assessment should be done before lung transplantation. In the Tokman et al. [194] series of 14 lung transplant recipients with telomerase mutations, renal disease, leukopenia prompting a change in the immunosuppressive regimen, and recurrent LTRI were common, however; the proportion of patients developed chronic lung allograft dysfunction (CLAD) was similar to other lung transplant patients. The systemic complications associated with telomerase dysfunction such as myelosuppression, cirrhosis, and malignancy may influence the outcome of successful lung transplant as the immunosuppressive drugs also possess myelosuppressive, hepatotoxic and carcinogenic effects [194]. In the series of Silhan et al. [193] dialysis was required post-transplant in 50% of patients. The authors suggested that nephrotoxic drugs used in the transplant setting may uncover a telomere-related renal vulnerability. Telomere shortening in patients with pulmonary fibrosis, particularly those with FPF, is a poor prognostic marker and portends a worse prognosis and increased morbidity after lung transplantation. In an observational cohort study done in sporadic IPF patients, telomere length was an independent predictor of transplant-free survival independent of age, sex, FVC, and diffusion capacity [195]. Telomere length <10th percentile for age is independently associated with worse survival and a shorter time to onset of chronic lung allograft dysfunction [195]. Therefore, telomere length may be used for risk stratification before lung transplantation. Smoking has a negative impact on patients with telomerase-related mutations. The average age of death in patients who are smokers and having telomerase-related mutations is 10 years earlier than that of non-smokers [165]. Lung transplantation in patients with ILD due to telomeropathy needs special attention. They may develop severe haematological complications, particularly after immunosuppressive therapy. The pre-transplant challenge with cytotoxic drugs may be used to test the robustness of bone marrow reserves, and to identify patients who can tolerate the haematological stress of transplant-related complications. Nephrotoxic drug such as Calcineurin inhibitors may uncover a telomere-related renal vulnerability [193]. Silhan et al. [193] proposed the following pre-transplant workup for patients suspected to have telomere syndrome; genetic counselling and evaluation, formal haematology consultation, consult with the experienced center regarding the feasibility of bone marrow challenge with myelotoxic drugs and assessment of liver parenchyma for subclinical evidence of cirrhosis.

9.7. Impact of Transplant

The outcome of lung transplantation in IPF patients with underlying telomerase mutations showed poor results in retrospective case series [192, 193, 194]. One retrospective cohort of nine patients from France showed that patients with telomerase mutations had an increased the risk of severe hematologic complications, in particular, bone marrow failure after lung transplantation with a post-transplant median survival of 214 days [192]. In the Tokman et al. [194] series of 14 lung transplant recipients with telomerase mutations, renal disease, leukopenia prompting a change in the immunosuppressive regimen, and recurrent LTRI were common, however; the proportion of patients developed chronic lung allograft dysfunction (CLAD) was similar to other lung transplant patients. The systemic complications associated with telomerase dysfunction such as myelosuppression, cirrhosis, and malignancy may influence the outcome of successful lung transplant as the immunosuppressive drugs also possess myelosuppressive, hepatotoxic and carcinogenic effects. Brestoff et al. [195] published a case report of acute graft-versus-host disease (GVHD) post lung transplant in a patient with underlying *TERT* mutation. Newman et al. [196] assessed the clinical outcome of lung transplant based on telomere length. Telomere length <10th percentile for age was detected in 32% of patients. They reported that a telomere length below 10th percentile for age was independently associated with a worse survival hazard ratio 10.9, 95% confidence interval 2.7–44.8, p = 0.001), a shorter time to onset of chronic lung allograft dysfunction (CLAD), (hazard ratio 6.3, 95% confidence interval 2.0–20.0, p = 0.002), but no increased risk for acute cellular rejection, infection, renal/hepatic disease/hematologic dysfunction.

Therefore, telomere length may be used for risk stratification before lung transplantation. Courtwright et al. recommend pre-transplant screening for short telomeres among ILD candidates be limited to the following subsets: individuals with a personal history of early graying (before 30 years old), cytopenias or macrocytosis, and/or abnormal liver function tests or imaging suggestive of hepatic impairment without other explanation; or with a family history of one or more first degree relatives with ILD. T cell depleting agents such as anti-thymocyte globulin should be avoided as ATG has been associated with increased telomere shortening and decreased telomerase activity in kidney transplant recipients [197]. Monitoring of renal, hepatic and bone marrow function post-transplant is warranted, particularly for recipients with *TERC* mutations, who appear to be at higher risk for bone marrow dysfunction [161]. Koppelstaetter et al. [198] had shown that calcineurin inhibitors, particularly cyclosporine may shorten telomeres more significantly than the mTOR inhibitor sirolimus. In patients with persistent cytopenias, mTOR inhibitors can be considered [199].

The efficacy and safety of antifibrotics in patients with IPF and associated telomerase mutations need to be studied prospectively. Justet et al. [200] in a small retrospective series reported that Pirfenidone was well-tolerated, however, failed to show improvement in FVC or DL_{CO} decline. Danazol, an androgenic synthetic sex hormone, was recently studied in 27 patients with telomere-related diseases (bone marrow failure and pulmonary fibrosis) [201]. The dose of Danazol given orally was 800 mg divided into two doses per day for a period of 2 years. Danazol caused elongation of telomere length and the effect was recorded as early as 6 months with a mean increase of 386 bp at 24 months. A positive hematological response was seen in 79% of cases. In the IPF subset, Danazol therapy had shown stabilization of diffusing capacity of the lung for carbon monoxide (DLCO), FVC and chest CT scan findings during the 2-year therapy. The main adverse effects are hepatotoxicity, muscle cramps and increased risk of venous thrombosis. However, still more conclusive evidence is available, use of Danazol should be restricted to patients with aplastic anemia [202]. The short telomere may explain the adverse outcome such as increased mortality, hospitalizations, and treatment-related severe adverse events seen in IPF patients treated with a combination of prednisone, azathioprine, and N-acetylcysteine in PANTHER-IPF clinical trial [203, 112]. Le Saux et al. [204] had shown a beneficial effect of telomerase activator, GRN510 in a mouse model with heterozygous *TERT* mutation with bleomycin-induced pulmonary fibrosis. It needs a human study to confirm this finding.

9.8. Pathogenesis

The mechanisms by which telomere defects initiate pulmonary fibrosis are not fully understood. Evidences are available linking defects in telomere maintenance with alveolar epithelial cell senescence, alveolar epithelial stem cell failure and an impaired response to epithelial injury [205, 206]. Epithelial senescence or apoptosis by stimulating a lung remodelling response may cause pulmonary fibrosis [207]. Snetselaar et al. had demonstrated a significantly shorter telomere length in AT2 cells in the fibrotic areas compared to the non-fibrotic areas, implicating telomere shortening within AT2 cells in the pathogenesis of IPF [173]. Another mechanism of action of *TERT* is via regulation of the Wnt–β-catenin pathway. The Wnt/β-catenin pathway is an important regulator of cellular proliferation and differentiation and abnormal activation of Wnt/β-catenin signal was observed in IPF [208, 209, 210]. The Wnt–β-catenin pathway promotes EMT and myofibroblast differentiation in vitro [211, 212]. In mouse embryonic stem cells and Wnt reporter mice, *TERT* can act as a transcriptional activator of Wnt signalling by complexing with β catenin [213].

10. GENES FOR EPITHELIAL INTEGRITY

These are the genes involved in cell-cell adhesion. Fingerlin et al. in a GWAS identified multiple susceptibility genes for fibrotic IIP and two of them includes desmoplakin (*DSP* at 6p24) and dipeptidyl peptidase 9 (DPP9 at 19p13) [26]. *DSP* is an obligate component of desmosomes and is responsible for maintaining epithelial cell-cell adhesion, wound healing and epithelial integrity [214, 215]. Fingerlin et al. [26] also showed that the lung tissue expression of *DSP* was significantly increased compared to controls (P = 0.0002), and the expression varied by genotype at *rs2076295* (P = 0.002). Mathai et al. [216] studied the association between *DSP* variants and IPF and the relationship of the variants with DSP gene expression in lung tissues. The intron 5 variant (*rs2076295*) is associated with an increased risk of IPF (odds ratio = 1.36, 95% CI = 1.19–1.56, P = 0.001) after adjusting age and gender. They also demonstrated a higher gene expression of *DSP* in IPF lung (p=0.0001). However, patients with IPF carrying the minor allele (G) at *rs2076295* variant was associated with a decreased gene expression of *DSP* in both IPF lung and control lung tissues. The GG genotype showed a 1.54-fold decrease (95% CI = 1.17–2.0, P = 0.002) in *DSP* expression compared with the TT genotype in IPF lungs. Immunostaining has shown localization of DSP to airway epithelia and not in alveolar tissue. This SNP indicates an aberrant repair of epithelial injury in IPF patient.

11. Chronic Hypersensitivity Pneumonitis

Non-IPF ILD such as CHP may have a genetic background. Okamoto in a Japanese cohort of 114 patients with a diagnosis of CHP identified familial clustering in 17.5% of cases [217]. Ley et al. [218] reported a significant association between *MUC5B* promoter variant *rs35705950* and short telomere length with fibrosis in patients with chronic hypersensitivity pneumonitis. Only the short telomere length <10th percentile for age was significantly associated with worse survival. However, neither the *MUC5B rs35705950* SNP nor the *TOLLIP rs5743890* SNP showed any association with survival.

12. CONNECTIVE TISSUE DISEASE-ASSOCIATED ILD (CTD-ILD)

Similar to IPF, CTD-ILD also develops due to the interaction between genes and environment. Fingerlin et al. [29] performed a genome-wide imputation-based association analysis among non-Hispanic whites with fibrotic idiopathic interstitial pneumonia (1,616 cases and 4,683 control subjects). They subsequently replicated their findings in an independent cohort (878 cases and 2,017 control subjects). They identified one novel locus in the HLA region of chromosome 6p21. (*rs7887* Pmeta = 3.7×10^{-09}) and two HLA alleles, DRB1*15:01 and DQB1*06:02, associated with fibrotic idiopathic interstitial pneumonia. Fingerlin et al. [29] also performed targeted RNA-sequencing of the HLA locus and identified 21 genes differentially expressed between fibrotic and control lung tissue, many of which play key roles in immune and inflammatory response regulation. These two alleles contribute to 35% variability at risk of fibrotic idiopathic interstitial pneumonias. Fibrotic interstitial pneumonia also includes several CTD-ILD such as scleroderma, rheumatoid arthritis, and systemic lupus erythematosus. Juge et al. [219] identified a shared genetic risk in patients with RA-ILD and FPF. In an exome-sequencing based study, they identified mutations linked to FPF in excess in RA-ILD patients (*TERT, RTEL1, PARN* or *SFTPC*). Familial aggregation similar to FPF had been detected in 25% of RA-ILD patients carrying at least one mutation in FPF-linked genes. RA-ILD patients with *TERT* or *RTEL1* mutations developed lLD earlier than those without mutations in telomerase-related genes, which may be due to anticipation. In another study, Juge et al. [220] evaluated the association between *MUC5B* promoter variant *rs35705950* in 620 patients with RA-ILD, 614 patients with RA without ILD, and 5448 unaffected controls and observed an increased risk of ILD among RA patients with *MUC5B* promoter variant. However; *MUC5B* promoter variant was not a risk factor for RA. The increased risk is specific for UIP radiological pattern only. Furukawa et al. [128] found that the DRB1*15 and DQB1*06 alleles have been associated with interstitial lung disease in a sample of rheumatoid arthritis patients in Japan, whereas the HLA-DRB1 shared epitopes was associated with a reduced risk of ILD. Newton et al. [221] also assessed the role of genomic markers in patients with interstitial pneumonia with autoimmune features (IPAF) and connective tissue disease-associated interstitial lung disease (CTD-ILD) with IPF as a comparator. In patients with IPAF, only *MUC5B rs35705950* and short telomere length were associated with worse survival and no association with survival was seen with the TOLLIP genotype. Neither short telomere length nor *MUC5B* mutations are associated with transplant-free survival among CTD-ILD patients.

13. GENE EXPRESSION

Selman et al. [222] conducted a microarray analysis on RNA extracted from lung tissues in 15 patients with IPF, 12 patients with CHP and eight patients with NSIP. The gene expression signatures were different in different ILDs, indicating different underlying pathogenetic mechanisms. Patients with IPF had upregulation of tissue remodelling, apoptosis, and fibroblast signalling genes, whereas, patients with CHP showed upregulation of genes associated with inflammation, T-cell activation, and immune responses. NSIP is more difficult to identify based on gene signature. Yang et al. [223] performed microarray analysis on peripheral blood RNA of 130 IPF patients and demonstrated that peripheral blood transcriptome can potentially differentiate normal individuals from patients with IPF. They can also distinguish the extent of IPF defined by DLco, but not when severity was categorized by percent predicted FVC. Gene expression profile may also help to identify the subgroup of patients with an accelerated course. Selman et al. [224] reported that the lungs of rapid progressors overexpressed genes involved in morphogenesis, oxidative stress, migration/proliferation, and fibrogenesis. The investigators verified two genes; adenosine-2B receptor and prominin-1/CD133. The adenosine-2B receptors are involved in lung fibroblasts differentiation [225]. BAL samples of rapid progressors group showed an increased in level of active

MMP-9 and a significantly higher fibroblast migration compared to slow progressors. Gene signature may also predict outcome in IPF patients. Herazo-Maya et al. [226] found that a 52-gene signature is a reproducible predictor of mortality and transplant-free survival in patients with IPF. The 52-gene signature when added to the Gender, Age, and Physiology (GAP) index significantly improved the performance of GAP index. Based on a genomic risk scoring system (Scoring Algorithm for Molecular Subphenotypes; SAMS), two risk groups were identified; low risk and high risk. Interestingly; untreated patients did not shift their risk profile over time, however, after the initiation of anti-fibrotic therapy, some high-risk patients had a reversal of their genomic risk profile. Therefore; the 52-gene expression profile may help in prognostication and disease monitoring. Steele et al. [227] studied gene expression profiling in 167 IIP lung tissues and 50 control lungs and its relation with lung function parameters. Interestingly; they found more commonalities than differences at gene expression level among different IIP subtypes, indicating that different subtypes may be related etiologically and pathogenically. However, they reported marked changes in expression of novel and established genes and pathways among progressive disease as measured by FVC and DLco. The rhotekin 2 (*RTKN2*), selecting E (*SELE*), and peptidase inhibitor 15 (*PI15*) were the gene transcripts most strongly associated with disease severity.

14. GENETIC TESTING

The 2011 ATS/ERS/JRS/ALAT guideline did not recommend genetic testing for IPF [5], however; the 2013 ATS/ERS statement on IIPs and French guidelines suggest genetic testing in FPF variety [228, 229]. Borie et al. [158] demonstrated no significant differences in the prevalence of disease-associated variant of *TERT/TERC* mutations between patients with FPF or patients with extra-pulmonary involvement suggestive of telomere syndrome features (18.2% versus 16.4%). Unlike the ATS/ERS statement on IIPs, French guideline 2018 [230] performing *TERT/TERC* sequencing in patients with extra-pulmonary signs. Initially, clinical and biological signs of genetic cause should be searched in all patients with IPF along with family history. The French 2018 guideline recommended searching for a genetic cause in the following subset of patients with IPF; the presence of a family history of ILD and clinical and biological evidence supporting a genetic cause (age < 50 years; hematological, hepatic or mucocutaneous abnormalities).

A thorough family history should be taken at baseline and during follow up visits also as up to 10% of patients diagnosed as "sporadic IPF" may have a family member diagnosed with an IIP during follow-up, sometimes many years later [231]. A personal or family history of cryptogenic cirrhosis, aplastic anemia, and/or premature graying of hair should also be elicited along with a family history of short-telomere. A PBMC telomere length <10% of age is a predictor of telomerase-related gene mutations. Wang et al. (73) demonstrated a link between SFTA2 mutation with FPF and Adenocarcinoma lung. Therefore, analysis of surfactant-related gene should be undertaken in patients with a family history of early-onset ILD with a history of lung cancer [231]. The genetic testing focussed primarily on the telomerase complex genes and the surfactant protein-C genes [232]. Mutation of the telomerase complex may increase the risk of severe haematological complication after lung transplantation [231]. Genetic testing for the telomere-related mutation before lung transplantation is definitely an important issue that needs an answer.

15. Epigenetic Pathways

Creditable evidence is available suggesting the role of noncoding RNAs (ncRNAs) mutations in ILD. Non coding RNAs (ncRNAs) have been extensively studied and validated to have differential expression in different disease conditions. The ncRNAs can be broadly categorized into small (19-30 nucleotide (nt) long for e.g., microRNA-miRNAS) and long (approximately 200 nt for e.g., long-noncoding RNA-lincRNAs) sized RNAs and cover approximately 98% of the human genome [232].

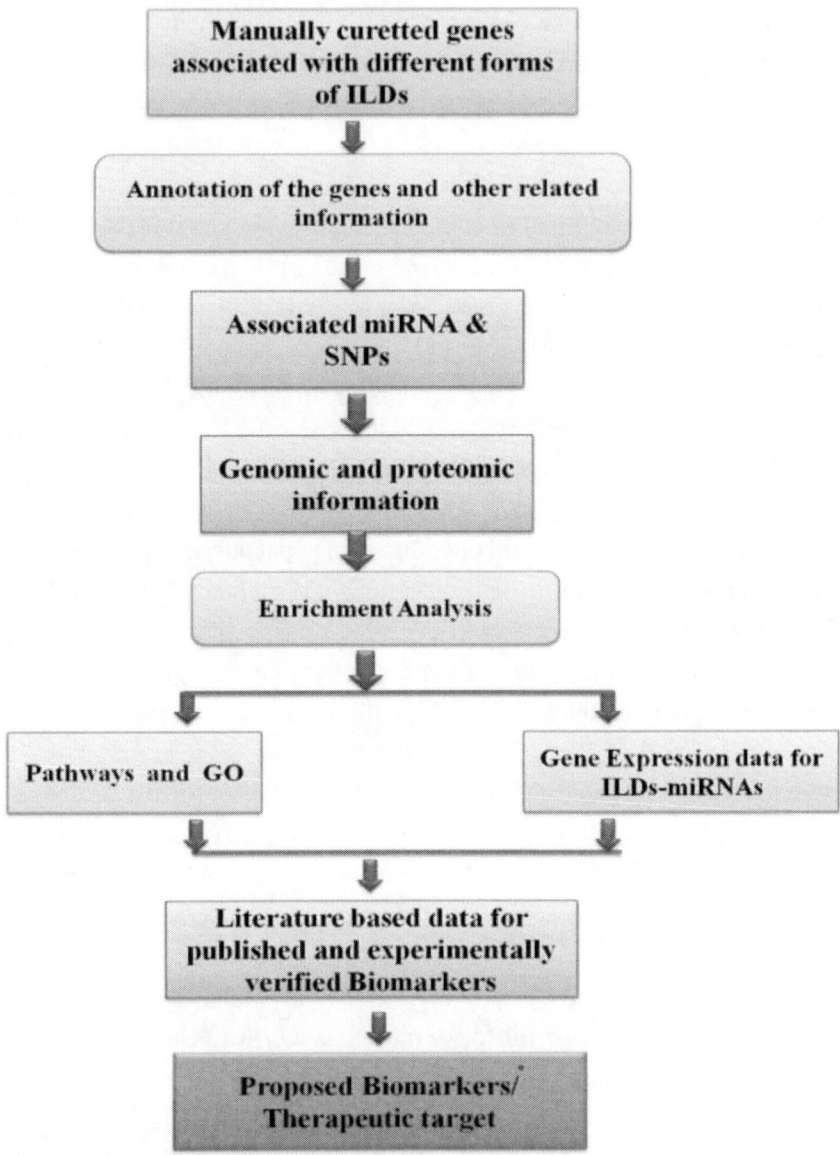

Figure 1. Showing a proposed pipeline for comprehensive analyses of miRNAs-lncRNAs-pathway associations with ILDs genes.

Role of these ncRNAs has been extensively studied as novel biomarkers and different therapeutic interventions [233]. In comparison with standard biomarkers, the biochemical nature of ncRNAs offers better stability and flexible storage conditions of the samples, and increased sensitivity and specificity [234]. The cross-regulation between miRNAs and lncRNAs towards competing endogenous RNAs (ceRNAs) activity are also significant for disease diagnosis and monitoring. Systematic investigation and analyses of these regulatory elements can provide potential biomarkers for ILDs [235]. Many analyses explored the role of these regulatory elements as therapeutic/biomarker targets, and outlines the biological functions, differential expression and pathways association of the most significant ncRNAs [236]. Many studies demonstrated the significant impact of ncRNAs and their target interactions to provide the new directions for ILDs diagnosis and monitoring through non-invasive interventions [237].

The reported outcomes from ongoing studies on ncRNAs-pathways and ceRNAs networks analysis provide clear insight to theorize that the ncRNAs influence molecular pathways, and can be key aspects in the etiology of ILDs. As discussed earlier, the ILDs are mainly immunologically-mediated diseases; therefore, miRNAs, lncRNAs and ceRNAs are expected to play an essential role in ILDs progression. However, only a few miRNAs are recognized as established biomarkers/therapeutic targets for ILDs subtypes [238]. The ncRNAs and their association with ILD-genes and pathways have significant implications in many ILDs (such as IPF and systemic sclerosis) pathogenesis and diagnostics [239]. Therefore, these interactions could be functionally characterized and verified for their vital role as ILDs genetic biomarkers. Considering these facts into account, a pipeline for comprehensive analyses of miRNAs-lncRNAs-pathway associations with ILDs genes has been proposed in Figure 1.

CONCLUSION

Interstitial lung diseases develop due to the interaction between gene and environment. Genetic studies have linked several common and rare genetic variants associated with ILD. There are data available showing strong and replicable associations between common and rare genetic variants and ILD. Genetical analysis in ILD has a potential role in early diagnosis also. These variants are involved in different pathogenic pathways which needs detailed exploration in the future. Elucidating the pathways linked to a particular gene has the potential for developing newer therapeutic options in the future. Genetics in ILD also helps in prognostication, phenotyping ILD, and deciding the therapeutics. Future clinical trials in ILD should also include genetic information for outcome analysis.

REFERENCES

[1] Antoniou, K. M., Margaritopoulos, G. A., Tomassetti, S., Bonella, F., Costabel, U., Poletti, V. 2014. "Interstitial lung disease." *European Respiratory Review* 23: 40-54.

[2] Cottin, V., Hirani, N. A., Hotchkin, D. L., et al. 2018. "Presentation, diagnosis and clinical course of the spectrum of progressive-fibrosing interstitial lung diseases." *European Respiratory Review* 27: 180076.

[3] Mira-Avendano, I., Abril, A., Burger, C. D., Dellaripa, P. F.,. Fischer, A., Gotway, M. B., Lee, A. S., Lee, J. S., Matteson, E. L., Yi, E. S., Ryu, J. H. 2019. "interstitial lung disease and other pulmonary manifestations in connective tissue diseases." *Mayo Clinic Proceedings* 94(2):309-325.

[4] Garantziotis, S., Steele, M. P., Schwartz, D. A. 2004. "Pulmonary fibrosis: thinking outside of the lung." *Journal of Clinical Investigation* 114:319–321.

[5] Raghu, G., Collard, H. R., Egan, J. J., Martinez, F. J., Behr, J., Brown, K. K., et al. 2011. "An official ATS/ERS/JRS/ALAT statement: idiopathic pulmonary fibrosis: evidence-based guidelines for diagnosis and management." *American journal of respiratory and critical care medicine* 183(6):788–824.

[6] Meltzer, E. B., Noble, P. W. 2008. "Idiopathic pulmonary fibrosis." *Orphanet Journal of Rare Diseases* 3:8.

[7] Marshall, R. P., McAnulty, R. J., Laurent, G. J. 1997. "The pathogenesis of pulmonary fibrosis: is there a fibrotic gene?" *The International Journal of Biochemistry and Cell Biology* 29:107–20.

[8] Marshall, R. P., Puddicombe, A., Cookson, W. O., Laurent, G. J. 2000. "Adult familial cryptogenic fibrosing alveolitis in the United Kingdom." *Thorax* 55(2):143-6.

[9] Ward, P. A., Hunninghake, G. W. 1998. "Lung inflammation and fibrosis." *American journal of respiratory and critical care medicine* 157:S123–S129.

[10] Dokal, I. 2000. "Dyskeratosis congenita in all its forms." *British Journal of Haematology* 110:768–79.

[11] Hermasnky, F, Pudlak, P. 1959. "Albinism associated with hemorrhagic diathesis and unusual pigmented reticular cells in the bone marrow. Report of two cases with histochemical studies." *Blood* 14:162.

[12] Auwrex, J., Demedts, M., Bouillon, R., et al. 1985. "Coexistence of hypocalcuric hypercalcaemia and interstitial lung disease in a family: a cross-sectional study." *European Journal of Clinical Investigation* 15:6-14.

[13] Riccardi, V. M. 1981. "Von Recklinghausen neurofibromatosis." *The New England Journal of Medicine* 305:1617-27.

[14] Harris, J. O., Waltuck, B. L., Swenson, E. W. 1969. "The pathophysiology of the lungs in tuberous sclerosis. A case report and literature review." *The American Review of Respiratory Diseases* 100:379-87.

[15] Schneider, E. L., Epstein, C. J., Kaback, M. J., et al. 1977. "Severe pulmonary involvement in adult Gaucher's disease. Report of three cases and review of the literature." *The American Journal of Medicine* 63:475-80.

[16] Sandoz, E. 1907. "A report of twins with fatal lung fibrosis, honeycomb lung and bronchiectasis [in German]." *Beitr Path Anat*, 41:495.

[17] Javaheri, S., Lederer, D. H., Pella, J. A., Mark, G. J., Levine, B. W. 1980. "Idiopathic pulmonary fibrosis in monozygotic twins: the importance of genetic predisposition." *Chest* 78:591-594.

[18] Solliday, N. H., Williams, J. A., Gaensler, E. A., Coutu, R. E., Carrington, C. 1973. "Familial chronic interstitial pneumonia." *The American Review of Respiratory Diseases* 108:193-204.

[19] Bonanni, P. P., Frymoyer, J. W., Jacox, R. F. 1965. "A family study of idiopathic pulmonary fibrosis: a possible dysproteinemic and genetically determined disease." *The American Journal of Medicine* 39:411-421.

[20] Lee, H. L., Ryu, J. H., Wittmer, M. H., Hartman, T. E., Lymp, J. F., Tazelaar, H. D., Limper, A. H. 2005. "Familial idiopathic pulmonary fibrosis: clinical features and outcome." *Chest* 127:2034–2041.

[21] Hodgson, U., Laitinen, T., Tukiainen, P. 2002. "Nationwide prevalence of sporadic and familial idiopathic pulmonary fibrosis: evidence of founder effect among multiplex families in Finland." *Thorax* 57:338–342.

[22] Swaye, P., van Ordstrand, H. S., McCormack, L. J., Wolpaw, S. E. 1969. "Familial Hamman-Rich syndrome." *Chest* 55:7–12.

[23] Kaur, A., Mathai, S. K., Schwartz, D. A. 2017. "Genetics in idiopathic pulmonary fibrosis pathogenesis, prognosis, and treatment." *Front Med (Lausanne)* 4:154.

[24] Chu, S. G., El-Chemaly, S., Rosas, I. O. 2016. "Genetics and Idiopathic Interstitial Pneumonias." *Seminar in Respiratory Critical Care Medicine* 37(3):321-30.

[25] Mushiroda, T., Wattanapokayakit, S., Takahashi, A., et al. 2008. "A genome-wide association study identifies an association of a common variant in TERT with susceptibility to idiopathic pulmonary fibrosis." *Journal of Medical Genetics* 45:654–56.

[26] Fingerlin, T. E., Murphy, E., Zhang, W., Peljto, A. L., Brown, K. K., Steele, M. P., Loyd, J. E., Cosgrove, G. P., Lynch, D., Groshong, S., et al. 2013. "Genome-wide association study identifies multiple susceptibility loci for pulmonary fibrosis." *Nature Genetics* 45(6):613–20.

[27] Noth, I., Zhang, Y., Ma, S. F., et al. 2013. "Genetic variants associated with idiopathic pulmonary fibrosis susceptibility and mortality: a genome-wide association study." *The Lancet Respiratory Medicine* 1:309–17.

[28] Codd, V., Nelson, C. P., Albrecht, E., et al. 2013. "Identification of seven loci affecting mean telomere length and their association with disease." *Nature Genetics* 45(4):422–427, e1–e2.

[29] Fingerlin, T. E., Zhang, W., Yang, I. V., Ainsworth, H. C., Russell, P. H., Blumhagen, R. Z., et al. 2016. "Genome-wide imputation study identifies novel HLA locus for pulmonary fibrosis and potential role for auto-immunity in fibrotic idiopathic interstitial pneumonia." *BMC Genetics* 17:74.

[30] Ennis, S. 2013. "IPF and chromosome 11p: lightning strikes twice?." *The Lancet Respiratory Medicine* 1(4):278-9.

[31] Allen, R. J., Porte, J., Braybrooke, R., Flores, C., Fingerlin, T. E., Oldham, J. M., et al. 2017. "Genetic variants associated with susceptibility to idiopathic pulmonary fibrosis in people of European ancestry: a genome-wide association study." *The Lancet Respiratory Medicine* 5:869–80.

[32] Moore, C., Blumhagen, R. Z., Yang, I. V., Walts, A., Powers, J., Walker, T., et al. 2019. "Resequencing study confirms host defense and cell senescence gene variants contribute to the risk of idiopathic pulmonary fibrosis." *American journal of respiratory and critical care medicine* Apr 29. doi: 10.1164/rccm.201810-1891OC. [Epub ahead of print].

[33] Hobbs, B. D., de Jong, K., Lamontagne, M., Bosse, Y., Shrine, N., Artigas, M. S., Wain, L. V., Hall, I. P., et al. 2017. "Genetic loci associated with chronic obstructive pulmonary disease overlap with loci for lung function and pulmonary fibrosis." *Nature Genetics* 49: 426-432.

[34] Van Moorsel, C. H., van Oosterhout, M. F., Barlo, N. P., et al. 2010. "Surfactant protein C mutations are the basis of a significant portion of adult familial pulmonary fibrosis in a Dutch cohort." *American journal of respiratory and critical care medicine* 182:1419–1425.

[35] García-Sancho, C., Buendía-Roldán, I., Fernández-Plata, M. R., Navarro, C., Pérez-Padilla, R., Vargas, M. H., Loyd, J. E., Selman, M. 2011. "Familial pulmonary fibrosis is the strongest risk factor for idiopathic pulmonary fibrosis." *Respiratory Medicine* 105:1902–1907.

[36] Loyd, J. E. 2013. "Pulmonary fibrosis in families." *American journal of respiratory cell and molecular biology* 29 (3, Suppl) S47–S50.

[37] Steele, M. P., Speer, M. C., Loyd, J. E., et al. 2005. "Clinical and pathologic features of familial interstitial pneumonia." *American journal of respiratory and critical care medicine* 172:1146–1152.

[38] Rosas, I. O., Ren, P., Avila, N. A., et al. 2007. "Early interstitial lung disease in familial pulmonary fibrosis." *American journal of respiratory and critical care medicine* 176 (7): 698-705.

[39] El-Chemaly S., Ziegler S. G., Calado R. T., et al. 2011. "Natural history of pulmonary fibrosis in two subjects with the same telomerase mutation." *Chest* 139:1203–1209.

[40] Diaz de Leon A., Cronkhite J. T., Yilmaz C., et al. 2011. "Subclinical lung disease, macrocytosis, and premature graying in kindreds with telomerase (TERT) mutations." *Chest* 140:753–763.

[41] Kropski, J. A., Blackwell, T. S., Loyd, J. E. 2015. "The genetic basis of idiopathic pulmonary fibrosis." *European Respiratory Journal* 45(6):1717–1727.

[42] Kropski, J. A., Pritchett, J. M., Zoz, D. F., et al. 2015. "Extensive phenotyping of individuals at risk for familial interstitial pneumonia reveals clues to the pathogenesis of interstitial lung disease." *American journal of respiratory and critical care medicine* 191(4):417–426.

[43] Johnston, I. D. A., Prescott, R. J., Chalmers, J. C., et al. 1997. "British Thoracic Society study of cryptogenic fibrosing alveolitis: current presentations and management." *Thorax* 52:38–44.

[44] Whitsett J. A., Wert S. E., Weaver T. E. 2010. "Alveolar surfactant homeostasis and the pathogenesis of pulmonary disease." *Annual Review of Medicine* 61:105–119.

[45] Maitra, M., Wang, Y., Gerard, R. D., Mendelson, C. R., Garcia, C. K. 2010. "Surfactant protein A2 mutations associated with pulmonary fibrosis lead to protein instability and endoplasmic reticulum stress." *The Journal of Biological Chemistry* 285(29):22103–22113.

[46] Perez-Gil, J., Weaver, T.E. 2010. "Pulmonary surfactant pathophysiology: current models and open questions." *Physiology (Bethesda)* 25(3):132-41.

[47] Beers, M. 1998. "Molecular processing and cellular metabolism of surfactant protein C. In: Rooney SA, editor. Lung surfactant: cellular and molecular processing." Austin: R.G. Landes. pp. 93–124.

[48] Johansson, J. 1998. "Structure and properties of surfactant protein C." *Biochimica et Biophysica Acta* 1408:161–172.

[49] Yamano, G., Funahashi, H., Kawanami, O., Zhao, L. X., Ban, N., Uchida, Y., Morohoshi, T., Ogawa, J., Shioda, S., Inagaki, N. 2001. "ABCA3 is a lamellar body membrane protein in human lung alveolar type II cells." *FEBS Letters* 508:221–225.

[50] Ban, N., Matsumura, Y., Sakai, H., Takanezawa, Y., Sasaki, M., Arai, H., Inagaki, N. 2007. "ABCA3 as a lipid transporter in pulmonary surfactant biogenesis." *The Journal of Biological Chemistry* 282:9628–9634.

[51] Glasser, S. W., Korfhagen, T. R., Weaver, T. E., Clark, J. C., Pilot-Matias, T., et al. 1998. "cDNA, deduced polypeptide structure and chromosomal assignment of human pulmonary surfactant proteolipid, SPL (pVal)." *The Journal of Biological Chemistry* 263:9–12.

[52] Sanchez-Pulido, L., Devos, D., Valencia, A. 2002. "BRICHOS: a conserved domain in proteins associated with dementia, respiratory distress and cancer." *Trends in Biochemical Sciences* 27:329–332.

[53] Mulugeta, S., Nguyen, V., Russo, S. J., Muniswamy, M., Beers, M. F. 2005. "A surfactant protein C precursor protein BRICHOS domain mutation causes endoplasmic reticulum stress, proteasome dysfunction, and caspase 3 activation." *American journal of respiratory cell and molecular biology* 32(6):521–530.

[54] Borie, R., Kannengiesser, C., Crestani, B. 2012. "Familial forms of nonspecific interstitial pneumonia/idiopathic pulmonary fibrosis:

clinical course and genetic background." *Current Opinion in Pulmonary Medicine* 18(5):455-61.

[55] Nogee, L. M., Dunbar, AE III., Wert, S. E., Askin, F., Hamvas, A., Whitsett, J. A. 2001. "A mutation in the surfactant protein C gene associated with familial interstitial lung disease." *The New England Journal of Medicine* 344:573–579.

[56] Thomas, A. Q., Lane, K., Phillips, J. 3rd., et al. 2002. "Heterozygosity for a surfactant protein C gene mutation associated with usual interstitial pneumonitis and cellular nonspecific interstitial pneumonitis in one kindred." *American journal of respiratory and critical care medicine* 165: 1322–1328.

[57] Fernandez, B. A., Fox, G., Bhatia, R., et al. 2012. "A Newfoundland cohort of familial and sporadic idiopathic pulmonary fibrosis patients: clinical and genetic features." *Respiratory Res*earch 13: 64.

[58] Coghlan, M. A., Shifren, A., Huang, H. J., et al. 2014. "Sequencing of idiopathic pulmonary fibrosis-related genes reveals independent single gene associations." *BMJ Open Respiratory Research* 1: e000057.

[59] Brasch, F., Griese, M., Tredano, M., Johnen, G., Ochs, M., Rieger, C., Mulugeta, S., Müller, K. M., Bahuau, M., Beers, M. F. 2004. "Interstitial lung disease in a baby with a de novo mutation in the SFTPC gene." *European Respiratory Journal* 24:30–39.

[60] Cameron, H. S., Somaschini, M., Carrera, P., Hamvas, A., Whitsett, J. A., Wert, S. E., Deutsch, G., Nogee, L. M. 2005. "A common mutation in the surfactant protein C gene associated with lung disease." *Journal of Pediatrics* 146 (3): 370-375.

[61] Crossno, P. F., Polosukhin, V. V., Blackwell, T. S., Johnson, J. E., Markin, C., Moore, P. E., Worrell, J. A., Stahlman, M. T., Phillips, J. A., Loyd, J. E., Cogan, J. D., Lawson, W. E. 2010. "Identification of early interstitial 658 lung disease in an individual with genetic variations in ABCA3 and SFTPC." *Chest* 137: 4: 969-973.

[62] Mechri, M., Epaud, R., Emond, S., et al. 2010. "Surfactant protein C gene (SFTPC) mutation-associated lung disease: high-resolution

computed tomography (HRCT) findings and its relation to histological analysis." *Pediatrics Pulmonology* 45:1021–1029.

[63] Cottin, V., Reix, P., Khouatra, C., Thivolet-Béjui, F., Feldmann, D., Cordier, J. F. 2011. "Combined pulmonary fibrosis and emphysema syndrome associated with familial SFTPC mutation." *Thorax* 66(10):918-9.

[64] Ono, S., Tanaka, T., Ishida, M., Kinoshita, A., Fukuoka, J., Takaki, M., et al. 2011. "Surfactant protein C G100S mutation causes familial pulmonary fibrosis in Japanese kindred." *European Respiratory Journal* 38(4):861-9.

[65] Lawson, W. E., Grant, S. W., Ambrosini, V., et al. 2004. "Genetic mutations in surfactant protein C are a rare cause of sporadic cases of IPF." *Thorax* 59: 977–980.

[66] Markart, P., Ruppert, C., Wygrecka, M., et al. 2007. "Surfactant protein C mutations in sporadic forms of idiopathic interstitial pneumonias." *European Respiratory Journal* 29: 134–137.

[67] Wang, W. J., Mulugeta, S., Russo, S. J., Beers, M. F. 2003. "Deletion of exon 4 from human surfactant protein C results in aggresome formation and generation of a dominant negative." *Journal of Cell Science* 116:683–692.

[68] Korfei, M., Ruppert, C., Mahavadi, P., et al. 2008. "Epithelial endoplasmic reticulum stress and apoptosis in sporadic idiopathic pulmonary fibrosis." *American journal of respiratory and critical care medicine 178*(8), 838–846.

[69] Hawkins, A., Guttentag, S.H., Deterding, R., Funkhouser, W.K., Goralski, J. L., Chatterjee, S., et al. 2015. "A non-BRICHOS SFTPC mutant (SP-CI73T) linked to interstitial lung disease promotes a late block in macroautophagy disrupting cellular proteostasis and mitophagy." *American journal of physiology. Lung cellular and molecular physiology 308*(1), L33–L47.

[70] Pardo, A. and Selman, M. 2002. "Idiopathic pulmonary fibrosis: new insights in its pathogenesis." *The International Journal of Biochemistry & Cell Biology* 34(12), 1534-1538.

[71] Zhong, Q., Zhou, B., Ann, D., Minoo, P., Liu, Y., Banfalvi, A., Krishnaveni, M., Dubourd, M., Demaio, L., Willis, B., Kim, K., duBois, R., Crandall, E., Beers, M. and Borok, Z. 2011. "Role of Endoplasmic Reticulum Stress in Epithelial–Mesenchymal Transition of Alveolar Epithelial Cells." *American Journal of Respiratory Cell and Molecular Biology* 45(3), 498-509.

[72] Lawson, W., Cheng, D., Degryse, A., Tanjore, H., Polosukhin, V., Xu, X., Newcomb, D., Jones, B., Roldan, J., Lane, K., Morrisey, E., Beers, M., Yull, F. and Blackwell, T. 2011. "Endoplasmic reticulum stress enhances fibrotic remodeling in the lungs." *Proceedings of the National Academy of Sciences*, 108(26), 10562-10567.

[73] Wang, Y., Kuan, P., Xing, C., Cronkhite, J., Torres, F., Rosenblatt, R., DiMaio, J., Kinch, L., Grishin, N. and Garcia, C. 2009. "Genetic Defects in Surfactant Protein A2 Are Associated with Pulmonary Fibrosis and Lung Cancer." *The American Journal of Human Genetics* 84(1), 52-59.

[74] Van Moorsel, C., ten Klooster, L., van Oosterhout, M., de Jong, P., Adams, H., Wouter van Es, H., Ruven, H., van der Vis, J. and Grutters, J. 2015. "SFTPA2Mutations in Familial and Sporadic Idiopathic Interstitial Pneumonia." *American Journal of Respiratory and Critical Care Medicine* 192(10): 1249-1252.

[75] Maitra, M., Wang, Y., Gerard, R., Mendelson, C. and Garcia, C. 2010. "Surfactant Protein A2 Mutations Associated with Pulmonary Fibrosis Lead to Protein Instability and Endoplasmic Reticulum Stress." *Journal of Biological Chemistry*, 285(29):22103-22113.

[76] Zhu, B., Ferry, C., Markell, L., Blazanin, N., Glick, A., Gonzalez, F. and Peters, J. 2014. "The Nuclear Receptor Peroxisome Proliferator-activated Receptor-β/δ (PPARβ/δ) Promotes Oncogene-induced Cellular Senescence through Repression of Endoplasmic Reticulum Stress." *Journal of Biological Chemistry* 289(29): 20102-20119.

[77] Nathan, N., Giraud, V., Picard, C., Nunes, H., Dastot-Le Moal, F., Copin, B., Galeron, L., De Ligniville, A., Kuziner, N., Reynaud-Gaubert, M., Valeyre, D., Couderc, L., Chinet, T., Borie, R., Crestani, B., Simansour, M., Nau, V., Tissier, S., Duquesnoy, P., Mansour-

Hendili, L., Legendre, M., Kannengiesser, C., Coulomb-L'Hermine, A., Gouya, L., Amselem, S. and Clement, A. 2016. "Germline SFTPA1mutation in familial idiopathic interstitial pneumonia and lung cancer." *Human Molecular Genetics* 25(8): 1457-1467.

[78] Beers, M. and Mulugeta, S. 2005. "Surfactant protein c biosynthesis and its emerging role in conformational lung disease." *Annual Review of Physiology* 67(1): 663-696.

[79] Mulugeta, S., Gray, J., Notarfrancesco, K., Gonzales, L., Koval, M., Feinstein, S., Ballard, P., Fisher, A. and Shuman, H. 2002. "Identification of LBM180, a Lamellar Body Limiting Membrane Protein of Alveolar Type II Cells, as the ABC Transporter Protein ABCA3." *Journal of Biological Chemistry* 277(25): 22147-22155.

[80] Wert, S., Whitsett, J. and Nogee, L. 2009. "Genetic Disorders of Surfactant Dysfunction." *Pediatric and Developmental Pathology* 12(4): 253-274.

[81] Shulenin, S., Nogee, L., Annilo, T., Wert, S., Whitsett, J. and Dean, M. 2004. "ABCA3Gene Mutations in Newborns with Fatal Surfactant Deficiency." *New England Journal of Medicine* 350(13): 1296-1303.

[82] Campo, I., Zorzetto, M., Mariani, F., Kadija, Z., Morbini, P., Dore, R., et al. 2014. "A large kindred of pulmonary fibrosis associated with a novel ABCA3 gene variant." *Respiratory Research* 15:43.

[83] Young, L. R., Nogee, L. M., Barnett, B., Panos, R. J., Colby, T. V., Deutsch, G. H. 2008. "Usual interstitial pneumonia in an adolescent with ABCA3 mutations." *Chest* 2008 134(1):192-5.

[84] Epaud, R., Delestrain, C., Louha, M., Simon, S., Fanen, P., Tazi, A. 2014. "Combined pulmonary fibrosis and emphysema syndrome associated with ABCA3 mutations." *European Respiratory Journal* 43(2): 638–641.

[85] Bullard, J. E., Nogee, L. M. 2007. "Heterozygosity for ABCA3 mutations modifies the severity of lung disease associatedwith a surfactant protein C gene (SFTPC) mutation." *Pediatric Research* 62(2):176–179.

[86] Kumar, A., Dougherty, M., Findlay, G. M., et al. 2014. "Genome sequencing of idiopathic pulmonary fibrosis in conjunction with a medical school human anatomy course." *PLoS One* 9(9):e106744.

[87] Fahy, J. V., Dickey, B. F. 2010. "Airway mucus function and dysfunction." *The New England Journal of Medicine* 363:2233–2247.

[88] Button, B., et al. 2012. "A periciliary brush promotes the lung health by separating the mucus layer from airway epithelia." *Science* 337:937–941.

[89] Williams, O. W., Sharafkhaneh, A., Kim, V., Dickey, B. F., Evans, C. M. 2006. "Airway mucus: From production to secretion." *American journal of respiratory cell and molecular biology* 34(5):527-36.

[90] Seibold, M. A., Wise, A. L., Speer, M. C., Steele, M. P., Brown, K. K., Loyd, J. E., Fingerlin, T. E., Zhang, W., Gudmundsson, G., Groshong, S. D., et al. 2011. "A common MUC5B promoter polymorphism and pulmonary fibrosis." *The New England Journal of Medicine* 364: 1503–12.

[91] Mathai, S. K., Yang, I. V., Schwarz, M. I., Schwartz, D. A. 2015. "Incorporating genetics into the identification and treatment of Idiopathic Pulmonary Fibrosis." *BMC Medicine* 13:191.

[92] Yang, I. V., Fingerlin, T. E., Evans, C. M., Schwarz, M. I., Schwartz, D. A. 2015. "MUC5B and Idiopathic Pulmonary Fibrosis." *Annals of the American Thoracic Society* 12 Suppl 2(Suppl 2):S193-9.

[93] Horimasu, Y., Ohshimo, S., Bonella, F., Tanaka, S., Ishikawa, N., Hattori, N., et al. 2015. "MUC5B promoter polymorphism in Japanese patients with idiopathic pulmonary fibrosis." *Respirology* 20:439–44.

[94] Stock, C. J., Sato, H., Fonseca, C., et al. 2013. "Mucin 5B promoter polymorphism is associated with idiopathic pulmonary fibrosis but not with development of lung fibrosis in systemic sclerosis or sarcoidosis." *Thorax* 68:436–441.

[95] Borie, R., Crestani, B., Dieude, P., Nunes, H., Allanore, Y., et al. 2013. "The MUC5B Variant Is Associated with Idiopathic pulmonary fibrosis but not with systemic sclerosis interstitial lung disease in the European Caucasian population." *PLoS ONE* 8(8): e70621.

[96] Plantier, L., Crestani, B., Wert, S. E., Dehoux, M., Zweytick, B., et al. 2011. "Ectopic respiratory epithelial cell differentiation in bronchiolised distal airspaces in idiopathic pulmonary fibrosis." *Thorax* 66: 651–657.

[97] Hunninghake, G. M., Hatabu, H., Okajima, Y., Gao, W., Dupuis, J., Latourelle, J. C., Nishino, M., et al. 2013. "MUC5B promoter polymorphism and interstitial lung abnormalities." *The New England Journal of Medicine* 368:2192–200.

[98] Araki, T., Putman, R. K., Hatabu, H., Gao, W., Dupuis, J., Latourelle, J. C., et al. 2016. "Development and progression of interstitial lung abnormalities in the Framingham Heart Study." *American journal of respiratory and critical care medicine* 194(12):1514–22.

[99] Peljto, A. L., Selman, M., Kim, D. S., Murphy, E., Tucker, L., Pardo, A., et al. 2015. "The MUC5B promoter polymorphism is associated with idiopathic pulmonary fibrosis in a Mexican cohort but is rare among Asian ancestries." *Chest* 147:460–464.

[100] Wang, C., Zhuang, Y., Guo, W., Cao, L., Zhang, H., Xu, L., Fan, Y., Zhang, D., Wang, Y. 2014. "Mucin 5B promoter polymorphism is associated with susceptibility to interstitial lung diseases in Chinese males." *PLoS One* 9:e104919.

[101] Peljto, A. L., Zhang, Y., Fingerlin, T. E., et al. 2013. "Association between the MUC5B promoter polymorphism and survival in patients with idiopathic pulmonary fibrosis." *JAMA* 309(21):2232-9.

[102] Cosgrove, G. P., Groshong, S. D., Peljto, A. L., et al. 2012. "The *MUC5B* promoter polymorphism is associated with a less severe pathological form of familial interstitial pneumonia (FIP) [abstract]." *American Journal of Respiratory and Critical Care Medicine* 185:A6865.

[103] Evans, C.M., Fingerlin, T.E., Schwarz, M.I., Lynch, D., Kurche, J., Warg, L., et al. 2016. "Idiopathic pulmonary fibrosis: a genetic disease that involves mucociliary dysfunction of the peripheral airways." *Physiological Reviews* 96:1567–1591.

[104] Nakano, Y., Yang, I. V., Walts, A. D., Watson, A. M., Helling, B. A., Fletcher, A. A., et al. 2016. "MUC5B promoter variant rs35705950

affects MUC5B expression in the distal airways in idiopathic pulmonary fibrosis." *American Journal of Respiratory and Critical Care Medicine* 193:464–466.

[105] Yang, I. V., Coldren, C. D., Leach, S. M., Seibold, M. A., Murphy, E., Lin, J., et al. 2013. "Expression of cilium-associated genes defines novel molecular subtypes of idiopathic pulmonary fibrosis." *Thorax* 68:1114–1121.

[106] Gharib, S. A., Altemeier, W. A., Van Winkle, L. S., et al. 2013. "Matrix metalloproteinase-7 coordinates airway epithelial injury response and differentiation of ciliated cells." *American Journal of Respiratory Cell and Molecular Medicine* 48:390–6.

[107] Boucher, R. C. 2011. "Idiopathic pulmonary fibrosis--a sticky business." *The New England Journal of Medicine* 364(16):1560-1.

[108] Chung, J. H., Peljto, A. L., Chawla, A., et al. 2016. "CT Imaging Phenotypes of Pulmonary Fibrosis in the MUC5B Promoter Site Polymorphism." *Chest* 149(5):1215-22.

[109] Bulut, Y., Faure, E., Thomas, L., Equils, O., Arditi, M. 2001. "Cooperation of Tolllike receptor 2 and 6 for cellular activation by soluble tuberculosis factor and *Borrelia burgdorferi* outer surface protein A lipoprotein: role of Toll-interacting protein and IL-1 receptor signalling molecules in Toll-like receptor 2 signaling." *Journal of Immunology* 167: 987–94.

[110] Zhu, L., Wang, L., Luo, X., et al. 2012. "Tollip, an intracellular trafficking protein, is a novel modulator of the transforming growth factor-beta signaling pathway." *The journal of biological chemistry* 287: 39653–63.

[111] Oldham, J. M., Ma, S. F., Martinez, F. J., et al. 2015. "TOLLIP, MUC5B, and the Response to N-Acetylcysteine among Individuals with Idiopathic Pulmonary Fibrosis." *American journal of respiratory and critical care medicine* 192(12):1475-82.

[112] Idiopathic Pulmonary Fibrosis Clinical Research Network, Raghu, G., Anstrom, K. J., King, T. E., Jr., Lasky, J. A., Martinez, F. J. 2012. "Prednisone, azathioprine, and N-acetylcysteine for pulmonary fibrosis." *The New England Journal of Medicine* 366: 1968-1977.

[113] Santiago, F. M., Bueno, P., Olmedo, C., Muffak-Granero, K., Comino, A., Serradilla, M., Mansilla, A., et al. 2008. "Effect of Nacetylcysteine administration on intraoperative plasma levels of interleukin-4 and interleukin-10 in liver transplant recipients." *Transplantation Proceedings* 40:2978–2980.

[114] O'Dwyer, D. N., Armstrong, M. E., Trujillo, G., et al. 2013. "The Toll-like receptor 3 L412F polymorphism and disease progression in idiopathic pulmonary fibrosis." *American journal of respiratory and critical care medicine* 188: 1442–1450.

[115] Hodgson, U., Pulkkinen, V., Dixon, M., Peyrard-Janvid, M., Rehn, M., Lahermo, P., et al. 2006. "ELMOD2 is a candidate gene for familial idiopathic pulmonary fibrosis." *The American Journal of Human Genetics* 79:149–54.

[116] Gumienny, T. L., Brugnera, E., Tosello-Trampont, A. C., Kinchen, J. M., Haney, L. B., Nishiwaki, K., et al. 2001. "CED-12/ELMO, a novel member of the crkII/Dock180/Rac pathway, is required for phagocytosis and cell migration." *Cell* 107, 27-41.

[117] Brugnera, E., Haney, L., Grimsley, C., Lu, M., Walk, S. F., Tosello-Trampont, A. C., Macara, I. G., Madhani, H., Fink, G. R., Ravichandran, K. S. 2002. "Unconventional Rac-GEF activity is mediated through the Dock180-ELMO complex." *Nature Cell Biology* 4, 574–582.

[118] DeBakker, C. D., Haney, L. B., Kinchen, J. M., Grimsley, C., Lu, M., Klingele, D., Hsu, P. K., et al. 2004. "Phagocytosis of apoptotic cells is regulated by a UNC-73/TRIO-MIG-2/RhoG signalling module and armadillo repeats of CED-12/ELMO." *Current Bioliogy* 14, 2208–221618.

[119] Pulkkinen, V., Bruce, S., Rintahaka, J., Hodgson, U., Laitinen, T., Alenius, H., et al. 2010. "ELMOD2, a candidate gene for idiopathic pulmonary fibrosis, regulates antiviral responses." *FASEB Journal* 24:1167–77.

[120] Erlich, H. A., Opelz, G., Hansen, J. 2001. "HLA DNA typing and transplantation." *Immunity* 14:347-56.

[121] Falfan-Valencia, R., Camarena, A., Juarez, A., Becerril, C., Montano, M., Cisneros, J., et al. 2005. "Major histocompatibility complex and alveolar epithelial apoptosis in idiopathic pulmonary fibrosis." *Human Genetics* 118:235-44.
[122] Zhang, J., Xu, D. J., Xu, K. F., Wu, B., Zheng, M. F., Chen, J. Y., et al. 2012. "HLA-A and HLA-B gene polymorphism and idiopathic pulmonary fibrosis in a Han Chinese population." *Respiratory Medicine* 106:1456-62.
[123] Xue, J., Gochuico, B. R., Alawad, A. S., Feghali-Bostwick, C. A., Noth, I., Nathan, S. D., et al. 2011. "The HLA class II Allele DRB1*1501 is overrepresented in patients with idiopathic pulmonary fibrosis." *PLoS One* 6:e14715.
[124] Fulmer, J. D., Sposovska, M. S., von Gal, E. R., Crystal, R. G., Mittal, K. K. 1978. "Distribution of HLA antigens in idiopathic pulmonary fibrosis." *American Reviews of Respiratory Diseases* 118:141-7.
[125] Turton, C. W., Morris, L. M., Lawler, S. D., Turner-Warwick, M. 1978. "HLA in cryptogenic fibrosing alveolitis." *Lancet* 1:507-8.
[126] Varpela, E., Tiilikainen, A., Varpela, M., Tukiainen, P. 1979. "High prevalences of HLA-B15 and HLA-Dw6 in patients with cryptogenic fibrosing alveolitis." *Tissue Antigens* 14:68-71.
[127] Falfan-Valencia, R., Camarena, A., Pineda, C. L., et al. 2014. "Genetic susceptibility to multicase hypersensitivity pneumonitis is associated with the TNF-238 GG genotype of the promoter region and HLADRB1* 04 bearing HLA haplotypes." *Respiratory Medicine* 108(1):211-217.
[128] Furukawa, H., Oka, S., Shimada, K., Sugii, S., Ohashi, J., Matsui, T., Ikenaka, T., Nakayama, H., Hashimoto, A., Takaoka, H., et al. 2012. "Association of human leukocyte antigen with interstitial lung disease in rheumatoid arthritis: a protective role for shared epitope." *PLoS One* 7(5), e33133.
[129] Aquino-Galvez, A., Pérez-Rodríguez, M., Camarena, A., Falfan-Valencia, R., Ruiz, V., Montaño, M., Barrera, L., Sada-Ovalle, I., et al. 2009. "MICA polymorphisms and decreased expression of the

MICA receptor NKG2D contribute to idiopathic pulmonary fibrosis susceptibility." *Human Genetics* 125(5-6):639-48.
[130] Selman, M., Pardo, A. 2006. "Role of epithelial cells in idiopathic pulmonary Wbrosis: from innocent targets to serial killers." *Proceedings of the American Thoracic Society* 3:364–372.
[131] Kim, K. K., Kugler, M. C., Wolters, P. J., Robillard, L., Galvez, M.G., Brumwell, A.N., Sheppard, D., Chapman, H.A. 2006. "Alveolar epithelial cell mesenchymal transition develops in vivo during pulmonary fibrosis and is regulated by the extracellular matrix." *Proceedings of the National Academy of Sciences of the United States of America* 103:13180–13185.
[132] Tamaki, S., Kawakami, M., Yamanaka, Y., Shimomura, H., Imai, Y., Ishida, J. I., Yamamoto, K., Ishitani, A., Hatake, K., Kirita, T. 2008. "Relationship between soluble MICA and the MICA A5.1 homozygous genotype in patients with oral squamous cell carcinoma." *Clinical Immunology* 130:331–337.
[133] Evans, C. 1976. "HLA antigens in diffuse fibrosing alveolitis." *Thorax* 31: 483–5.
[134] Strimlan, C. V., Taswell, H. F., DeRemee, R. A., Kueppers, F. 1977. "HLA antigens and fibrosing alveolitis." *The American Reviews of Respiratory Diseases* 1120–1.
[135] Zhang, H. P., Zou, J., Xie, P., Gao, F., Mu, H. J. 2015. "Association of HLA and cytokine gene polymorphisms with idiopathic pulmonary fibrosis." *Kaohsiung Journal of Medical Science* 31(12):613-20.
[136] Dinarello, C. A. 1996. "Biologic basis for interleukin-1 in disease." *Blood* 87:2095–2147.
[137] Nicklin, M. J., Weith, A., Duff, G. W. 1994. "A physical map of the region encompassing the human interleukin-1 alpha, interleukin-1 beta, and interleukin-1 receptor antagonist genes." *Genomics* 19:382–384.
[138] Whyte, M., Hubbard, R., Meliconi, R., et al. 2000. "Increased risk of fibrosing alveolitis associated with interleukin-1 receptor antagonist and tumor necrosis factor-alpha gene polymorphisms." *American*

journal of respiratory and critical care medicine 162(2, Pt 1):755–758.

[139] Barlo, N. P., vanMoorsel, C. H., Korthagen, N. M., et al. 2011. "Genetic variability in the IL1RN gene and the balance between interleukin (IL)-1 receptor agonist and IL-1β in idiopathic pulmonary fibrosis." *Clinical & Experimental Immunology* 166(3):346–351.

[140] Korthagen, N. M., van Moorsel, C. H., Kazemier, K. M., Ruven, H. J., Grutters, J. C. 2012. "IL1RN genetic variations and risk of IPF: a meta-analysis and mRNA expression study." *Immunogenetics* 64:371–7.

[141] Fernandez, I. E., Eickelberg, O. 2012. "The Impact of TGF-b on lung fibrosis from targeting to biomarkers." *Proceedings of the American Thoracic Society* 9(3):111–116.

[142] Son, J. Y., Kim, S. Y., Cho, S. H., Shim, H. S., Jung, J. Y., Kim, E. Y., Lim, J. E., Park, B. H., et al. 2013. "TGF-beta1 T869C polymorphism may affect susceptibility to idiopathic pulmonary fibrosis and disease severity." *Lung* 191:199–205.

[143] Xaubet, A., Marin-Arguedas, A., Lario, S., Ancochea, J., Morell, F., Ruiz-Manzano, J., Rodriguez-Becerra, E., Rodriguez-Arias, J. M., et al. 2003. "Transforming growth factor-beta1 gene polymorphisms are associated with disease progression in idiopathic pulmonary fibrosis." *American journal of respiratory and critical care medicine* 168:431–5.

[144] Pardo, A., Selman, M. 2012. "Role of matrix metaloproteases in idiopathic pulmonary fibrosis." *Fibrogenesis & Tissue Repair* 5(Suppl 1):S9.

[145] Pardo, A., Selman, M., Kaminski, N. 2008. "Approaching the degradome in idiopathic pulmonary fibrosis." *The International Journal of Biochemistry & Cell Biology* 40:1141-1455.

[146] Zuo, F., Kaminski, N., Eugui, E., Allard, J., Yakhini, Z., Ben-Dor, A., Lollini, L., Morris, D., Kim Y, et al. 2002. "Gene expression analysis reveals matrilysin as a key regulator of pulmonary fibrosis in mice and humans." *Proceedings of the National Academy of Sciences of the United States of America* 99:6292-97.

[147] Checa, M., Ruiz, V., Montaño, M., Velázquez-Cruz, R., Selman, M., Pardo, A. 2008. "MMP-1 polymorphisms and the risk of idiopathic pulmonary fibrosis." *Human Genetics* 124(5):465–472.

[148] Kong, C. M., Lee, X. W., Ang, W. X. 2013. "Telomere shortening in human diseases." *FEBS J* 280:3180–93.

[149] Zhao, Y., Sfeir, A. J., Zou, Y., Buseman, C. M., Chow, T. T., Shay, J. W. & Wright, W. E. 2009. "Telomere extension occurs at most chromosome ends and is uncoupled from fill-in in human cancer cells." *Cell* 138,463-75.

[150] d'Adda di Fagagna, F. 2008. "Living on a break: cellular senescence as a DNA damage response." *Nature Reviews Cancer* 8(7):512–22.

[151] Greider, C. W., Blackburn, E. H. 1985. "Identification of a specific telomere terminal transferase activity in Tetrahymena extracts." *Cell* 43:405-13.

[152] Mitchell, J. R., Wood, E., Collins, K. 1999. "A telomerase component is defective in the human disease dyskeratosis congenital." *Nature* 402:551–55.

[153] Chen, J. L., Blasco, M. A., Greide, C. W. 2000. "Secondary structure of vertebrate telomerase RNA." *Cell* 100:503–14.

[154] Podlevsky, J. D., Chen, J. J. L. 2012. "It all comes together at the ends: Telomerase structure, function, and biogenesis." *Mutation Research* 730:3-11

[155] Cong, Y. S., Wright, W. E., Shay, J. W. 2002. "Human telomerase and its regulation." *Microbiology and Molecular Biology Reviews* 2002; 66:407–25.

[156] Knight, S. W., Heiss, N. S., Vulliamy, T. J., et al. 1999. "X-linked dyskeratosis congenita is predominantly caused by missense mutations in the DKC1 gene." *The American Journal Human Genetics* 65(1):50–58.

[157] Vulliamy, T., Marrone, A., Goldman, F., Dearlove, A., Bessler, M., Mason, P. J., Dokal, I. 2001. "The RNA component of telomerase is mutated in autosomal dominant dyskeratosis congenital." *Nature* 413(6854):432-5.

[158] Raphael, B., Tabèze, L., Thabut, G., Nunes, H., Cottin, V., et al. 2016. "Prevalence and characteristics of TERT and TERC mutations in suspected genetic pulmonary fibrosis." *European Respiratory Journal* 48 (6):1721–31.

[159] Diaz de Leon, A., Cronkhite, J. T., Katzenstein, A. L., et al. 2010. "Telomere lengths, pulmonary fibrosis and telomerase (*TERT*) mutations." *PLoS One* 5: e10680.

[160] Armanios, M. 2009. "Syndromes of telomere shortening." *Annual Review of Genomics and Human Genetics* 10:45–61.

[161] Newton, C. A., Batra, K., Torrealba, J., Kozlitina, J., Glazer, C. S., Aravena, C., et al. 2016. "Telomere-related lung fibrosis is diagnostically heterogeneous but uniformly progressive." *European Respiratory Journal* 48(6):1710–20.

[162] Vulliamy, T., Marrone, A., Szydlo, R., Walne, A., Mason, P. J., Dokal, I. 2004. "Disease anticipation is associated with progressive telomere shortening in families with dyskeratosis congenita due to mutations in TERC." *Nature Genetics* 36(5):447–9.

[163] Cronkhite, J. T., Xing, C., Raghu, G., Chin, K. M., Torres, F., Rosenblatt, R. L., et al. 2008. "Telomere shortening in familial and sporadic pulmonary fibrosis." *American journal of respiratory and critical care medicine* 178(7):729–37.

[164] Kannengiesser, C., Borie, R., Renzoni, E. A. 2019. "Pulmonary fibrosis: Genetic analysis of telomere-related genes, telomere length measurement-or both?" *Respirology* 24(2):97-98.

[165] Tsakiri, K. D., Cronkhite, J. T., Kuan, P. J., et al. 2007. "Adult-onset pulmonary fibrosis caused by mutations in telomerase." *Proceedings of the National Academy of Sciences of the United States of America* 104:7552–7557.

[166] Alder, J. K., Chen, J. J. L., Lancaster, L., Danoff, S., Su, S., Cogan, J. D., et al. 2008. "Short telomeres are a risk factor for idiopathic pulmonary fibrosis." *Proceedings of the National Academy of Sciences of the United States of America* 105(35):13051–6.

[167] Armanios, M. 2012. "Telomerase and idiopathic pulmonary fibrosis." *Mutation Research* 730: 52–58.

[168] Armanios, M., Chen, J. L., Chang, Y. P., Brodsky, R. A., Hawkins, A., Griffin, C. A., Eshleman, J. R., Cohen, A. R., et al. 2005. "Haploinsufficiency of telomerase reverse transcriptase leads to anticipation in autosomal dominant dyskeratosis congenital." *Proceedings of the National Academy of Sciences of the United States of America* 102:15960–4.

[169] Armanios, M. Y., Chen, J. J., Cogan, J. D., et al. 2007. "Telomerase mutations in families with idiopathic pulmonary fibrosis." *The New England Journal of Medicine* 356:1317–1326.

[170] Parry, E. M., Alder, J. K., Qi, X., Chen, J. J. & Armanios, M. 2011. "Syndrome complex of bone marrow failure and pulmonary fibrosis predicts germline defects in telomerase." *Blood* 117, 5607–5611.

[171] Collopy, L. C., Walne, A. J., Cardoso, S., et al. 2015. "Triallelic and epigenetic-like inheritance in human disorders of telomerase." *Blood* 126: 176–184.

[172] Alder, J. K., Cogan, J. D., Brown, A. F., et al. 2011. "Ancestral mutation in telomerase causes defects in repeat addition processivity and manifests as familial pulmonary fibrosis." *PLoS Genetics* 7:e1001352.

[173] Snetselaar, R., van Batenburg, A. A., van Oosterhout, M. F. M., Kazemier, K. M., Roothaan, S. M., Peeters, T., et al. 2017. "Short telomere length in IPF lung associates with fibrotic lesions and predicts survival." *PLoS ONE* 12(12): e0189467.

[174] Planas-Cerezales, L., Arias-Salgado, E. G., Buendia-Roldán, I., Montes-Worboys, A., López, C. E., Vicens-Zygmunt, V., Hernaiz, P. L., Sanuy, R. L., et al. 2019. "Predictive factors and prognostic effect of telomere shortening in pulmonary fibrosis." *Respirology* 24(2):146-153.

[175] George, G., Rosas, I. O., Cui, Y., McKane, C., Hunninghake, G. M., Camp, P. C., et al. 2015. "Short telomeres, telomeropathy, and subclinical extrapulmonary organ damage in patients with interstitial lung disease." *Chest* 147:1549-1557.

[176] Chambers, D. C., Clarke, B. E., McGaughran, J., Garcia, C. K. 2012. "Lung Fibrosis, Premature Graying and Macrocytosis." *American*

Journal of Respiratory and and Critical Care Medicine 186(5): e8–e9.

[177] Stuart B. D., Choi J., Zaidi S., et al. 2015. "Exome sequencing links mutations in PARN and RTEL1 with familial pulmonary fibrosis and telomere shortening." *Nature Genetics* 47(5):512-517.

[178] Vannier, J. B., Sarek, G., Boulton, S. J. 2014. "RTEL1: functions of a disease-associated helicase." *Trends in Cell Biology* 24: 416-425.

[179] Vannier, J. B., Pavicic-Kaltenbrunner, V., Petalcorin, M. I., Ding, H., Boulton, S. J. 2012. "RTEL1 dismantles T loops and counteracts telomeric G4-DNA to maintain telomere integrity." *Cell* 149: 795-806.

[180] Cogan, J. D., Kropski, J. A., Zhao, M., Mitchell, D. B., Rives, L., Markin, C., Blackwell, T. S. 2015. "Rare variants in RTEL1 are associated with familial interstitial pneumonia." *American journal of respiratory and critical care medicine 191*(6): 646–655.

[181] Kannengiesser, C., Borie, R., Menard, C., Reocreux, M., Nitschke, P., Gazal, S., Mal, H., Taille, C., et al. 2015. "Heterozygous RTEL1 mutations are associated with familial pulmonary fibrosis." *European Respiratory Journal* 46: 474-485.

[182] Deng, Z., Glousker, G., Molczan, A., et al. 2013. "Inherited mutations in the helicase RTEL1 cause telomere dysfunction and Hoyeraal-Hreidarsson syndrome." *Proceedings of the National Academy of Sciences of the United States of America* 110(36):E3408–E3416.

[183] Borie, R., Bouvry, D., Cottin, V., Gauvain, C., Cazes, A., Debray, M.P., Cadranel, J., Dieude, P., et al. 2019. "Regulator of telomere length 1 (*RTEL1*) mutations are associated with heterogeneous pulmonary and extra-pulmonary phenotypes." *European Respiratory Journal* 53(2).

[184] Dressen, A., Abbas, A. R., Cabanski, C., et al. 2018. "Analysis of protein-altering variants in telomerase genes and their association with *MUC5B* variant status in patients with idiopathic pulmonary fibrosis: a candidate gene sequencing study." *The Lancet Respiratory Medicine* 6(8):603-614.

[185] Alder, J. K., Stanley, S. E., Wagner, C. L., Hamilton, M., Hanumanthu, V. S., & Armanios, M. 2014. "Exome sequencing identifies mutant TINF2 in a family with pulmonary fibrosis." *Chest* 147(5), 1361–1368.

[186] Frank, A. K., Tran, D. C., Qu, R. W., Stohr, B. A., Segal, D. J., Xu, L. 2015. "The shelterin TIN2 subunit mediates recruitment of telomerase to telomeres." *PLoS Genetics* 11(7):e1005410.

[187] Fukuhara, A., Tanino, Y., Ishii, T., et al. 2013. "Pulmonary fibrosis in dyskeratosis congenita with TINF2 gene mutation." *European Respiratory Journal* 42(6):1757–1759.

[188] Petrovski, S., Todd, J. L., Durheim, M. T., Wang, Q., Chien, J. W., Kelly, F. L., Goldstein, D. B. 2017. "An Exome Sequencing Study to Assess the Role of Rare Genetic Variation in Pulmonary Fibrosis." *American journal of respiratory and critical care medicine* 196(1), 82–93.

[189] Moon, D. H., Segal, M., Boyraz, B., Guinan, E., Hofmann, I., Cahan, P., Tai, A. K., Agarwal, S. 2015. "Poly(a)-specific ribonuclease (parn) mediates 3'-end maturation of the telomerase RNA component." *Nature genetics* 47:1482-1488.

[190] Coghlan, M. A., Shifren, A., Huang, H. J., et al. 2014. "Sequencing of idiopathic pulmonary fibrosis-related genes reveals independent single gene associations." *BMJ Open Respiratory Research* 1: e000057.

[191] Ley, B., Collard, H. R., King, TE Jr. 2011. "Clinical course and prediction of survival in idiopathic pulmonary fibrosis." *American Journal of Respiratory and Critical Care Medicine article* 183: 431–440.

[192] Borie, R., Kannengiesser, C., Hirschi, S., Le Pavec, J., Mal, H., et al. 2015. "Severe hematologic complications after lung transplantation in patients with telomerase complex mutations." *The Journal of Heart and Lung Transplantation* 34 (4), 538-546.

[193] Silhan, L. L., Shah, P. D., Chambers, D. C., Snyder, L. D., Riise, G. C., Wagner, C. L., et al. 2014. "Lung transplantation in telomerase

mutation carriers with pulmonary fibrosis." *European Respiratory Journal* 44(1):178–87.

[194] Tokman, S., Singer, J. P., Devine, M. S., Westall, G. P., Aubert, J. D., Tamm, M., et al. 2015. "Clinical outcomes of lung transplant recipients with telomerase mutations." *The Journal of Heart and Lung Transplantation* 34(10):1318–24.

[195] Brestoff, J. R., Vessoni, A. T., Brenner, K. A., Uy, G. L., DiPersio, J. F., Blinder, M., et al. 2018. "Acute graft-versus host disease following lung transplantation in a patient with a novel TERT mutation." *Thorax* 73:489-492.

[196] Newton, C. A., Kozlitina, J., Lines, J. R., Kaza, V., Torres, F., Garcia, C. K. 2017."Telomere length in patients with pulmonary fibrosis associated with chronic lung allograft dysfunction and post–lung transplantation survival." *The Journal of Heart and Lung Transplantation* 36:845-853.

[197] Crepin, T., Carron, C., Roubiou, C., Gaugler, B., Gaiffe, E., Simula-Faivre, D., *et al.* 2015. "ATG-induced accelerated immune senescence: Clinical implications in renal transplant recipients." *American Journal of Transplantation* 15:1028-1038.

[198] Koppelstaetter, C., Kern, G., Leierer, G., Mair, S. M., Mayer, G., Leierer, J. 2018. "Effect of cyclosporine, tacrolimus and sirolimus on cellular senescence in renal epithelial cells." *Toxicol In Vitro* 48:86-92.

[199] Courtwright, A. M., El-Chemaly, S. 2019. "Telomeres in Interstitial Lung Disease: The Short and the Long of It." *Annals of the American Thoracic Society* 16(2):175-181.

[200] Justet, A., Thabut, G., Manali, E., et al. 2018. "Safety and efficacy of pirfenidone in patients carrying telomerase complex mutation." *European Respiratory Journal* 51: 1701875.

[201] Townsley, D. M., Dumitriu, B., Liu, D., Biancotto, A., Weinstein, B., Chen, C., et al. 2016. "Danazol treatment for telomere diseases." *The New England Journal of Medicine* 374(20):1922–31.

[202] clinicaltrials.gov. Low-dose danazol for the treatment of telomere related diseases. NCT03312400; [accessed 2019, May 16th]. Available from: https://clinicaltrials.gov/ct2/show/NCT03312400.

[203] Newton, C. A., Zhang, D., Oldham, J. M., Kozlitina, J., Ma, S. F., Martinez, F. J., Raghu, G., Noth, I., Garcia, C. K. 2018. "Telomere length and use of immunosuppressive medications in idiopathic pulmonary fibrosis." *American Journal of Respiratory and Critical Care Medicine* article in press.

[204] Le Saux, C. J., Davy, P., Brampton, C., Ahuja, S. S., Fauce, S., et al. 2013. "A novel telomerase activator suppresses lung damage in a murine model of idiopathic pulmonary fibrosis." *PLoS ONE* 8(3): e58423.

[205] Alder, J. K., Barkauskas, C. E., Limjunyawong, N., Stanley, S. E., Kembou, F., Tuder, R. M., Hogan, B. L., Mitzner, W., Armanios, M. 2015. "Telomere dysfunction causes alveolar stem cell failure." *Proceedings of the National Academy of Sciences of the United States of America* 112:5099-5104.

[206] Kropski, J. A., Lawson, W. E., Young, L. R., Blackwell, T. S. 2013. "Genetic studies provide clues on the pathogenesis of idiopathic pulmonary fibrosis." *Disease models & mechanisms* 6:9-17.

[207] Alder, J. K., Guo, N., Kembou, F., Parry, E. M., Anderson, C. J., Gorgy, A. I., et al. 2011. "Telomere length is a determinant of emphysema susceptibility." *American Journal of Respiratory and Critical Care Medicine* 183, 904–12.

[208] Chilosi, M., Poletti, V., Zamò, A., Lestani, M., Montagna, L., Piccoli, P., Pedron, S., Bertaso, M., Scarpa, A., Murer, B. et al. 2003. "Aberrant Wnt/beta-catenin pathway activation in idiopathic pulmonary fibrosis." *The American Journal of Pathology* 162, 1495-1502.

[209] Königshoff, M., Balsara, N., Pfaff, E. M., Kramer, M., Chrobak, I., Seeger, W. and Eickelberg, O. 2008. Functional Wnt signaling is increased in idiopathic pulmonary fibrosis. *PLoS ONE* 3, e2142.

[210] Königshoff, M., Kramer, M., Balsara, N., Wilhelm, J., Amarie, O. V., Jahn, A., Rose, F., Fink, L., Seeger, W., Schaefer, L. et al. 2009.

"WNT1-inducible signalling protein-1 mediates pulmonary fibrosis in mice and is upregulated in humans with idiopathic pulmonary fibrosis." *Journal of Clinical Investigation* 119, 772-787.

[211] Carthy, J. M., Garmaroudi, F. S., Luo, Z. and McManus, B. M. 2011. "Wnt3a induces myofibroblast differentiation by upregulating TGF-β signaling through SMAD2 in a β-catenin-dependent manner." *PLoS ONE* 6, e19809.

[212] Zhou, B., Liu, Y., Kahn, M., Ann, D. K., Han, A., Wang, H., Nguyen, C., Flodby, P., Zhong, Q., Krishnaveni, M. S. et al. 2012. "Interactions between β-catenin and transforming growth factor-β signaling pathways mediate epithelial-mesenchymal transition and are dependent on the transcriptional co-activator cAMPresponse element-binding protein (CREB)-binding protein (CBP)." *The Journal of Biological Chemistry* 287, 7026-7038.

[213] Park, J. I., Venteicher, A. S., Hong, J. Y., Choi, J., Jun, S., Shkreli, M., Chang, W., Meng, Z., Cheung, P., Ji, H. et al. 2009. "Telomerase modulates Wnt signalling by association with target gene chromatin." *Nature* 460, 66-72.

[214] Ou, J., Lowes, C., Collinson, J. M. 2010. "Cytoskeletal and cell adhesion defects in wounded and Pax6$^{+/-}$ corneal epithelia." *Investigative Ophthalmology & Visual Science* 51:1415–1423.

[215] Al-Jassar, C., Bikker, H., Overduin, M., & Chidgey, M. 2013. "Mechanistic basis of desmosome-targeted diseases." *Journal of molecular biology*, 425(21), 4006–4022.

[216] Mathai, S. K., Pedersen, B. S., Smith, K., Russell, P., Schwarz, M. I., Brown, K.K., et al. 2016. "Desmoplakin Variants Are Associated with Idiopathic Pulmonary Fibrosis." *American Journal of Respiratory and Critical Care Medicine* 193(10):1151-60.

[217] Okamoto, T., Miyazaki, Y., Tomita, M., et al. 2013. "A familial history of pulmonary fibrosis in patients with chronic hypersensitivity pneumonitis." *Respiration* 85: 384–390.

[218] Ley, B., Newton, C. A., Arnould, I., Elicker, B. M., Henry, T. S., Vittinghoff, E., et al. 2017. "The MUC5B promoter polymorphism and telomere length in patients with chronic hypersensitivity

pneumonitis: an observational cohort-control study." *The lancet Respiratory medicine* 5(8):639-47.
[219] Juge, P. A., Borie, R., Kannengiesser, C., et al. 2017. "Shared genetic predisposition in rheumatoid arthritis-interstitial lung disease and familial pulmonary fibrosis." *European Respiratory Journal* 49(5).
[220] Juge, P. A., Lee, J. S., Ebstein, E., et al. 2018. "MUC5B promoter variant and rheumatoid arthritis with interstitial lung disease." *The New England Journal of Medicine* 2018;379(23):2209-2219.
[221] Newton, C. A., Oldham, J. M., Ley, B., et al. 2019. "Telomere Length and Genetic Variant Associations with Interstitial Lung Disease Progression and Survival." *European Respiratory Journal* 11;53(4).
[222] Selman, M., Pardo, A., Barrera, L., Estrada, A., Watson, S. R., Wilson, K., et al. 2006. "Gene expression profiles distinguish idiopathic pulmonary fibrosis from hypersensitivity pneumonitis." *American Journal of Respiratory and Critical Care Medicine* 173:188–98.
[223] Yang, I. V., Luna, L. G., Cotter, J., Talbert, J., Leach, S. M., Kidd, R., et al. 2012. "The peripheral blood transcriptome identifies the presence and extent of disease in idio-pathic pulmonary fibrosis." *PLoS One* 7:e37708.
[224] Selman, M., Carrillo, G., Estrada, A., Mejia, M., Becerril, C., Cisneros, J., et al. 2007. "Accelerated variant of idiopathic pulmonary fibrosis: clinical behavior and gene expression pattern." *PLoS One* 2:e482.
[225] Zhong, H., Belardinelli, L., Maa, T., Zeng, D. 2005. "Synergy between A2B adenosine receptors and hypoxia in activating human lung fibroblasts." *American Journal of Respiratory and Critical Care Medicine* 32: 2–8.
[226] Herazo-Maya, J. D., Sun, J., Molyneaux, P. L., Li, Q., Villalba, J. A., Tzouvelekis, A., et al. 2017. "Validation of a 52-gene risk profile for outcome prediction in patients with idiopathic pulmonary fibrosis: an international, multicentre, cohort study." *The Lancet Respiratory medicine* 5(11):857–868.

[227] Steele, M. P., Luna, L. G., Coldren, C. D., et al. 2015. "Relationship between gene expression and lung function in Idiopathic Interstitial Pneumonias." *BMC Genomics* 2015;16:869.
[228] Travis, W. D., Costabel, U., Hansell, D. M., et al. 2013. "An official American Thoracic Society/European Respiratory Society statement: Update of the international multidisciplinary classification of the idiopathic interstitial pneumonias." *American Journal of Respiratory and Critical Care Medicine* 188: 733–748.
[229] Cottin, V., Crestani, B., Valeyre, D., et al. 2014. "Diagnosis and management of idiopathic pulmonary fibrosis: French practical guidelines." *Eur Respir Rev* 23: 193–214.
[230] Cottin, V., Crestani, B., Cadranel, J., Cordier, J. F., Marchand-Adam, S., Prévot, G., et al. 2017. "French practical guidelines for the diagnosis and management of idiopathic pulmonary fibrosis – 2017 update." *Revue Des Maladies Respiratoires* 34(8), 900–968.
[231] Kropski, J. A., Young, L. R., Cogan, J. D., Mitchell, D. B., Lancaster, L. H., Worrell, J. A., Markin, C., Liu, N., Mason, W. R., Fingerlin, T. E., et al. 2017. "Genetic evaluation and testing of patients and families with idiopathic pulmonary fibrosis." *American Journal of Respiratory and Critical Care Medicine* 195:1423–1428.
[232] Carninci, P., Hayashizaki, Y. 2007. "Noncoding RNA transcription beyond annotated genes." *Current Opinion in Genetics & Development* 17:139–144.
[233] Van Roosbroeck, K., Pollet, J., Calin, G. A. 2013. "miRNAs and long noncoding RNAs as biomarkers in human diseases." *Expert review of molecular diagnostics* 13(2):183-204.
[234] Stępień, E., Costa, M. C., Kurc, S., Drożdż, A., Cortez-Dias, N., Enguita, F. J. 2018. "The circulating non-coding RNA landscape for biomarker research: lessons and prospects from cardiovascular diseases." *Acta Pharmacologica Sinica* 39(7):1085-1099.
[235] Kupczyk M., Kuna P. 2014. "MicroRNAs—new biomarkers of respiratory tract diseases." *Advances in Respiratory Medicine* 82(2):183-90.

[236] Chen T., He P., Tan Y, Xu D. 2017. "Biomarker identification and pathway analysis of preeclampsia based on serum metabolomics." *Biochemical and Biophysical Research Communications* 485(1):119-25.

[237] Mishra S., Shah M. I., Sarkar M., Asati N., Rout C. 2018. "ILDgenDB: integrated genetic knowledge resource for interstitial lung diseases (ILDs)." *Database*, 1–12.

[238] Lawson W. E., Blackwell T. S. and Gauldie J. 2011. "Let It Be: microRNAs impact interstitial lung disease." *Am J Respir Crit Care Med* 183:1-2.

[239] O'Reilly, S. 2016. "Epigenetics in Fibrosis." *Mol Aspects Med* 54, 89-102.

In: Interstitial Lung Disease
Editor: Liva T. Villadsen

ISBN: 978-1-53616-246-2
© 2019 Nova Science Publishers, Inc.

Chapter 2

IMAGING OF ACUTE INFILTRATIVE LUNG DISEASE

Meriem Affes* MD, Henda Nèji MD, Monia Attia MD, Saoussen Hantous-Zannad MD, Ines Baccouche MD, Jammoussi Amira MD and Khaoula Ben Miled-M'rad MD

Abderrahmen Mami Hospital, Ariana, Tunisia
Faculty of Medicine of Tunis, Tunis El Manar University,
Tunis, Tunisia

ABSTRACT

Acute infiltrative lung disease (AILD) is a heterogeneous group of lung disorders characterized by diffuse parenchymal lung involvement. It consists of an infiltrate of the interstitial lung tissue and/or distal airways (alveoli and respiratory bronchioles) which mainly occurs within 2 weeks and does not exceed one month. This group of infiltrative lung diseases

---

* Corresponding Author's: Meriem Affes - Imaging Department, Abderrahmen Mami Hospital, Ariana, Tunisia - Faculty of Medicine of Tunis, Tunis El Manar University, Tunis, Tunisia; Email: af_meriem@yahoo.fr.

may correspond to five histopathological presentations: diffuse alveolar damage, diffuse alveolar hemorrhage, immunoallergic pneumonia, acute organizing pneumonia and acute eosinophilic pneumonia. Each nosological entity may result from several causes. Moreover, the same disorder may have different histopathological manifestations.

AILD may result from many conditions. The main pathological causes are infections (bacterial, viral, fungal or parasitic) and hemodynamic overload (left ventricular failure). Cardiogenic pulmonary edema is easily suggested in the majority of cases on a chest CT scan. Typically, it is made up of regular septal thickening, "ground glass" opacities and consolidations associated with cardiomegaly, left atrium and pulmonary vein enlargement. Infections could be suggested in particular clinical conditions associated with *biologic inflammatory syndrome*. A bronchoalveolar lavage (BAL) is very useful, in this case, for the etiological diagnosis (pneumocystis, viruses...).

In addition to these common conditions, other rare causes have to be considered: acute respiratory distress syndrome, acute hypersensitivity pneumonitis, exposure to toxic gases and drugs including heroin or cocaine, connective tissue disease, or vasculitis which most often presents with alveolar hemorrhage. Acute Idiopathic organized pneumonia and acute idiopathic eosinophilic pneumonia are exclusion diagnoses.

A chest CT scan remains an essential examination in the assessment of AILD. A surgical pulmonary biopsy is unusual in the acute context. First of all, CT is useful in choosing the most suitable site for the BAL. It can suggest the cause in many cases. Semiological analysis of elementary lesions should be integrated with clinical data and the results of the BAL. There are different elementary patterns of AILD on CT scans including "ground glass" opacities, consolidations, septal thickening and micronodules. Their distribution as well as the predominant elementary lesions are helpful for diagnosis.

Keywords: computed tomography, lung, diffuse acute infiltrative lung disease, respiratory failure

INTRODUCTION

Acute infiltrative lung disease (AILD) is a heterogeneous group of lung disorders characterized by diffuse parenchymal lung involvement. It consists of an infiltrate of the interstitial lung tissue and/or distal airways (alveoli and respiratory bronchioles) which mainly occurs within 2 weeks and does not exceed one month. This group of infiltrative lung diseases may correspond to five histopathological presentations as a result of several different causes.

AILD may result from many conditions. The main pathological causes are infections and hemodynamic overload. Infections could be suggested in particular clinical conditions. Abronchoalveolar lavage (BAL) is very useful, in this case, for etiological diagnosis.

In addition to these common conditions, other rare causes have to be considered: acute hypersensitivity pneumonitis, exposure to toxic gases and drugs, connective tissue disease, or vasculitis which most often presents with alveolar hemorrhage. Acute Idiopathic organised pneumonia and acute idiopathic eosinophilic pneumonia are exclusion diagnoses.

A chest CT scan is a crucial examination in assessing AILD. A surgical pulmonary biopsy is unusual in the acute context. CT is useful in choosing the most suitable site for the BAL and in suggesting the cause in many cases. Semiological analysis of elementary lesions should be integrated with clinical data and the results of the BAL. There are different elementary patterns of AILD on CT scans including "ground glass" opacities (GGO), consolidations, septal thickening and micronodules. Their distribution as well as the predominant elementary lesions are helpful in suggesting the diagnosis.

1. CLASSIFICATION

AILD may correspond to five pathological entities: diffuse alveolar damage (DAD), diffuse alveolar hemorrhage (DAH), acute immunoallergic pneumonia (AIAP), acute organizing pneumonia (AOP) and acute eosinophilic pneumonia (AEP).

It should be known that this classification remains theoretical, and it is sometimes difficult to apply in practice.

In some cases, a CT scan can suggest the nature of this AILD and assign it to a pathological entity. However, it can sometimes be difficult to classify the observed condition based only on CT scan findings since the same elementary lesions can be found in several histopathological entities.

1.1. Diffuse Alveolar Damage (DAD)

Diffuse alveolar damage is the most frequently encountered finding in AILD.

1.1.1. Histology

It is characterized by two evolving phases: an exudative phase and a fibroproliferative one. The initial exudative phase develops during the first week after a pulmonary aggression and is characterized by the predominance of interstitial edema. Alveolar hemorrhage and hyaline membranes can also be noted. The second fibroproliferative phase is a repair one developing from the second week and is characterized by the proliferation of pneumocytes II and fibroblasts. Traction bronchiectasis and bronchiolectasis can be seen in the late fibrotic phase (Feuillet and Tazi 2011, Ichikado 2014).

1.1.2. Computed Tomography

There is a perfect correlation between histological phases and the CT features. The exudative phase is characterized by alveolitis and alveolar filling, which manifest mainly by GGO and consolidations with diffuse or patchy distribution (Figure 1). In the fibroproliferative phase, there is evidence of fibrosis attested mainly by bronchial distortion.

1.1.3. Etiologies

DAD is often associated with acute respiratory distress syndrome (ARDS). It may be seen in several conditions, mainly in infections, acute interstitial pneumonia (AIP) as well as organ and bone marrow recipients (Parambil et al. 2007).

1.2. Diffuse Alveolar Hemorrhage (DAH)

DAH corresponds to the extravasation of blood from the pulmonary acini micro-circulation, and not from the bronchial one, resulting in alveolar filling and affecting all the lungs homogeneously (Collard and Schwarz 2004).

1.2.1. Histology

DAH is attested to by the accumulation of red blood cells in the alveoli associated with fibrin and hemosiderin deposits in the alveolar walls. Hemosiderin-laden alveolar macrophages can also be noted. However, the most specific sign is capillaritis, which is reliable for positively diagnosing DAH and eliminating differential diagnoses including traumatic alveolar hemorrhage (resulting from surgical biopsy) (Collard and Schwarz 2004).

1.2.2. Computed Tomography

On a CT scan, the diagnosis of DAH is easily suggested in the presence of an underlying disease. Otherwise, the diagnosis can sometimes be difficult to make because of the nonspecific appearance of DAH on CT scans. Classically, it is made up of GGO with a central distribution that may be associated with consolidations with air bronchograms (Figure 2). In the subacute stage, septal thickening can be noted leading to a "crazy paving" appearance.

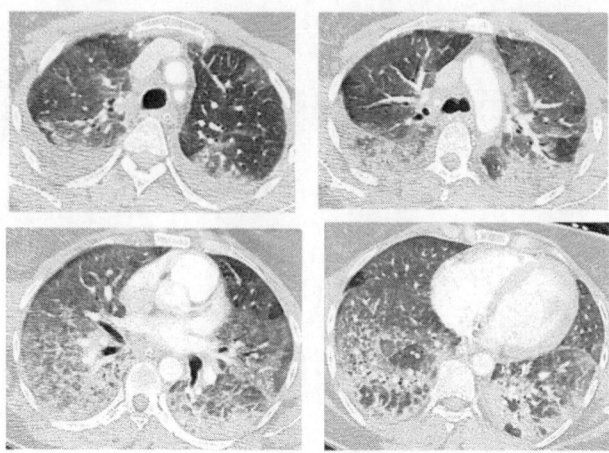

Figure 1. High-resolution CT findings corresponding to exudative phase of DAD with consolidations, patchy "ground-glass" opacities and focal spared areas. No bronchiectasis is observed.

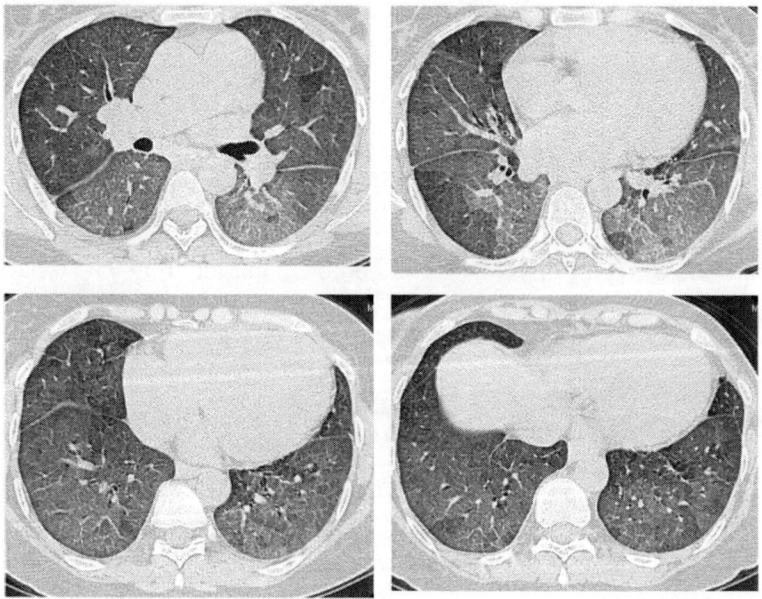

Figure 2. Chest CT scan with lung windowing in acute alveolar hemorrhage: Diffuse «ground glass» opacities.

1.2.3. Etiologies

Several conditions can lead to DAH. The main causes are ANCA vasculitis and Good Pasture syndrome (Figure 3). Connective tissue diseases can also be the cause, particularly systemic lupus erythematosus (Cordier 2006). Infections especially leptospirosis (Figure 4), toxic (cocaine) drugs (Propylthiouracile) and severe bleeding disorders may also be incriminated (Traclet et al. 2013).

1.3. Acute Organizing Pneumonia (AOP)

It is a form of inflammatory and fibroproliferative response of the pulmonary parenchyma to any aggression with a particular histological definition.

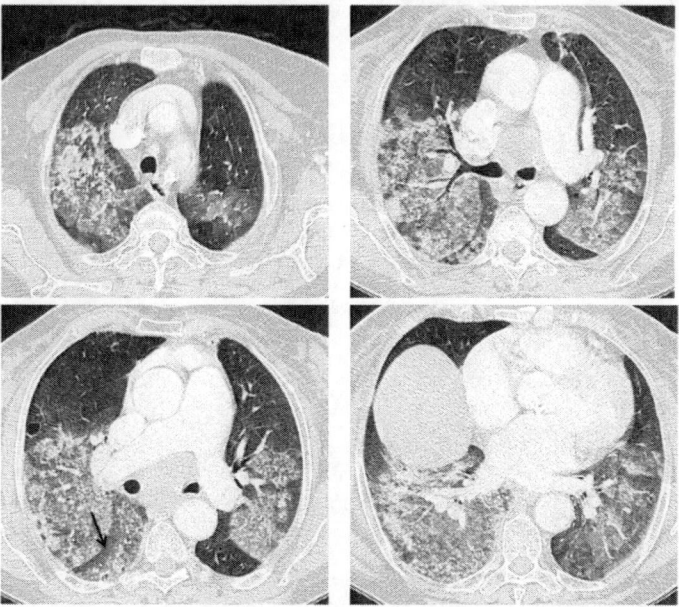

Figure 3. Chest CT with lung windowing during alveolar hemorrhage due to microscopic polyangiitis. Bilateral increasing lung attenuations with consolidations and « ground glass » opacities associated with septal thickening. Note the relative sparing of the extreme subpleural regions (arrow).

1.3.1. Histology

AOP is characterized by distal air spaces filled up with inflammatory cells, fibroblasts and myofibroblasts within a sparse extracellular matrix.

1.3.2. Computed Tomography

The typical appearance is made up of GGOs and consolidations with air bronchograms which may be dilated and distorted. Consolidations are often subpleural or peribronchovascular. The atoll sign, with central GGO and peripheral consolidation, is suggestive of the diagnosis but is not a specific pattern.

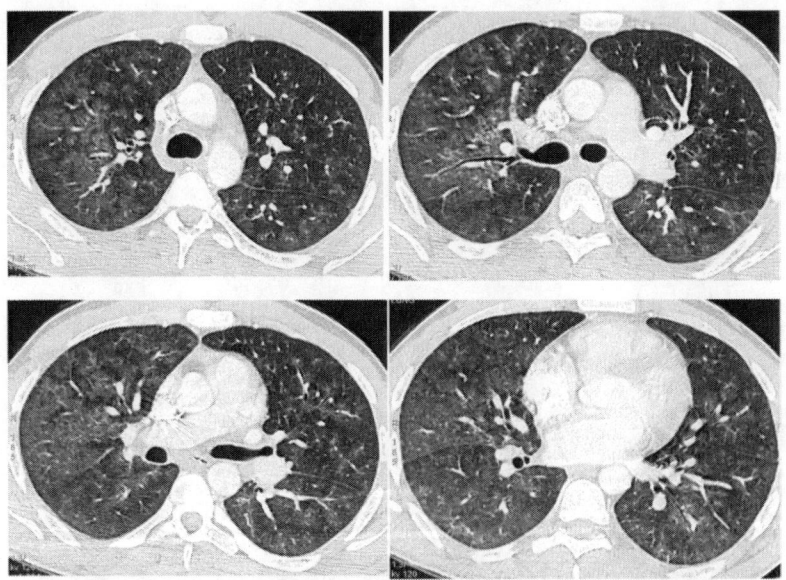

Figure 4. Diffuse alveolar hemorrhage due to leptospirosis in a 23-year-old man. CT scan shows bilateral patchy and centrilobular "ground-glass" attenuation.

1.3.3. Etiologies

AOP may be the result of drug intake, infection, or connective tissue disease. Sometimes no cause is found and AOP is considered idiopathic.

1.4. Acute Immunoallergic Pneumonia (AIAP)

Immunoallergic pneumonia, also named hypersensitivity pneumonia, is a hypersensitivity reaction of the lung in response to exposure of an inhaled antigen, most often an organic dust. Despite the term "hypersensitivity", this entity is not associated with atopy. Blood and alveolar eosinophils rates are normal (Franks and Galvin 2010).

Acute forms of immunoallergic pneumonia are due to a high level of exposure to an antigen over a short time. Symptoms develop within few hours and may include fever, chills, myalgia, fatigue, dyspnea and a non-productive cough. Once exposure ceases, recovery can be expected within a few days (KNUTSEN et al. 2019).

1.4.1. Histology

Microscopic observation shows a systematic presence of organizing pneumonia associated with poorly defined granulomas and interstitial lymphocyte infiltrate.

1.4.2. Computed Tomography

A chest CT scan typically shows GGO in AIAP, which is generally a nonspecific finding. It represents cellular interstitial infiltration, small granulomas within the alveolar septa, or both. These opacities may be found either centrally or peripherally, predominantly in the lower lung zones with apices sparing. This distribution is the opposite of the subacute or chronic hypersensitivity pneumonia which predominates to the upper and mid lungs. In the acute stage, there are neither reticulations nor signs of fibrosis in contrast to subacute and chronic forms (KNUTSEN et al. 2019).

1.4.3. Etiologies

There are more than 200 pathogens that can be responsible for acute hypersensitivity pneumonitis. They can be divided into four main groups: animal proteins, chemicals and drugs, bacteria, and fungi (KNUTSEN et al. 2019).

1.5. Acute Eosinophilic Pneumonia (AEP)

AEP is a rare disorder characterized by a rapid accumulation of eosinophils in the lungs. A positive diagnosis is based on a set of regularly revised criteria. Modified Philit criteria are currently used to diagnose AEP:

- Acute respiratory illness of less than 1 month
- Diffuse Infiltrative pneumonia on imaging
- BAL fluid eosinophilic rate more than 25% (or eosinophilic pneumonia on lung biopsy)
- Absence of other specific pulmonary eosinophilic diseases, including eosinophilic granulomatosis with polyangiitis (Churg-Strauss syndrome, hypereosinophilic syndrome, and allergic bronchopulmonary aspergillosis).

1.5.1. Histology

Histologic findings include marked interstitial and alveolar space infiltration with eosinophils associated with features of diffuse alveolar damage (hyaline membranes, fibroblast proliferation, and inflammatory cells). Airway mucus plugging and non-necrotic perivascular inflammation can occasionally be seen (Allen 2006).

1.5.2. Computed Tomography

AEP typically presents with GGO and patchy distributed consolidations with no particular predominance. Smooth septal thickening can be noted with possible "crazy paving" areas. Centrilobular nodules have been reported (Daimon et al. 2008). Rarely, peribronchial thickening can be noted (Figure 5). Bilateral pleural effusion is often associated.

There is no cardiomegaly which helps exclude acute cardiogenic edema (Daimon et al. 2008).

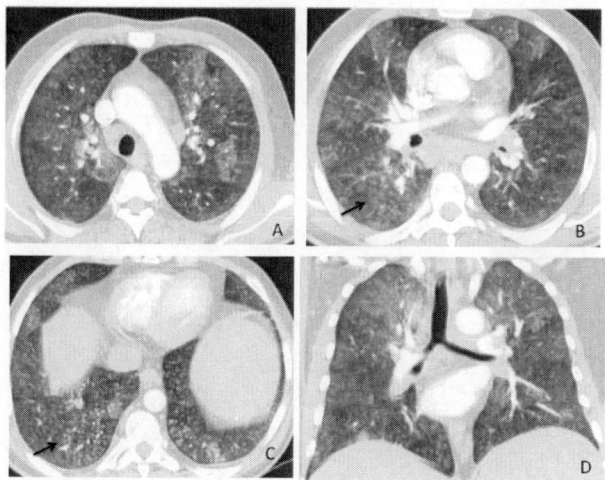

Figure 5. Acute eosinophilic pneumonia in a man. Axial CT images (A, B and C) and coronal reconstruction (D) demonstrate patchy "ground glass" opacities associated with poorly defined centrilobular nodules (arrows).

1.5.3. Etiologies

Acute eosinophilic pneumonia is most commonly idiopathic. Recent studies have reported multiple causes for AEP including tobacco smoke and other inhalants, drugs, and infection (parasitic and fungal infections). Tobacco smoking has been the most frequently implicated trigger in recent years (De Giacomi et al. 2018).

2. Etiological Forms

2.1. Infections

Infection is one of the most common causes of acute lung injury. Common bacteria rarely cause AILD. The most common pathogens are intracellular bacteria (mycoplasma pneumonia, legionella, mycobacteria), mycoses, viruses (influenza, RSV, CMV, and so on), and parasites (pneumocystosis, toxoplasmosis). Their radiological features are nonspecific, which explains the difficulty in identifying the causative organism. In spite of that, a meticulous analysis can sometimes guide the diagnosis, especially in pneumocystosis, which often gives rather suggestive radiological features.

2.1.1. Pneumocystosis

It is the most common opportunistic infection in immunocompromised patients, not only those infected with the human immunodeficiency virus (HIV), but also in subjects with lymphoproliferative syndrome as well as organ or hematopoietic stem cell recipients.

This infection is caused by *Pneumocystis Jirovecii* (previously known as Pneumocystis Carinii) which is a ubiquitous opportunistic fungus. CT can guide the diagnosis in many cases, but a positive diagnosis is based on BAL which makes it possible to detect cysts and trophozoites of P. *Jirovecii* (Lacombe et al. 2007).

Computed Tomography

A CT scan shows an AILD mainly made up of GGO associated with crazy paving and cysts. Areas of GGO may have geographical limits. It may also be diffuse or confluent. A reticular pattern and septal thickening are less frequent and may be due to either pulmonary edema or septal inflammatory cell infiltration (Figure 6). Pulmonary cysts, although highly suggestive, are noted in only 10 to 30% of cases (Lacombe et al. 2007, Marchiori et al. 2005). They can lead to a poorly tolerated pneumothorax because of its association with parenchymal involvement (Lacombe et al. 2007). Rarely, consolidation or micronodules can be noted. In this context, nodules are the radiological manifestation of granulomas which may, in rare cases, undergo necrosis and become excavated (Marchiori et al. 2005) (Figure 7). This AILD has a more or less bilateral symmetrical distribution with predominance in the upper lobes and with relative sparing of the subpleural regions (Figure 8). Under treatment, the evolution is often favorable without sequelae but fibrotic signs can sometimes be seen such as irregular septal thickening, traction bronchiectasis and architectural lung distortion (Marchiori et al. 2005, Lacombe et al. 2007).

Imaging of Acute Infiltrative Lung Disease

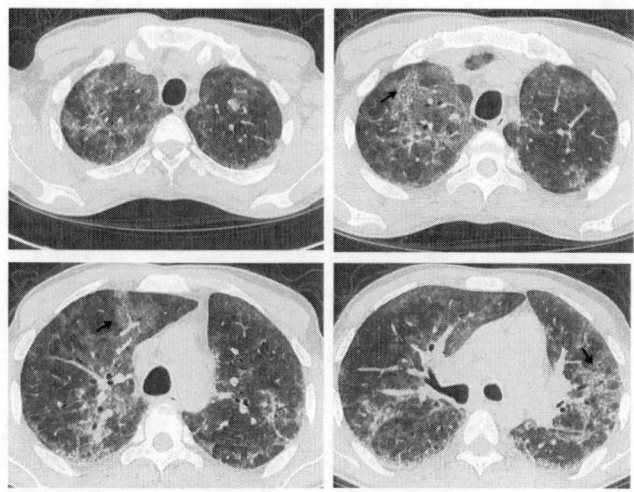

Figure 6. 37-year-old man with Hodgkin Lymphoma and pneumocystosis. High-resolution CT scan shows patchy bilateral ground glass opacities, small foci of consolidation, and a crazy paving pattern (arrows).

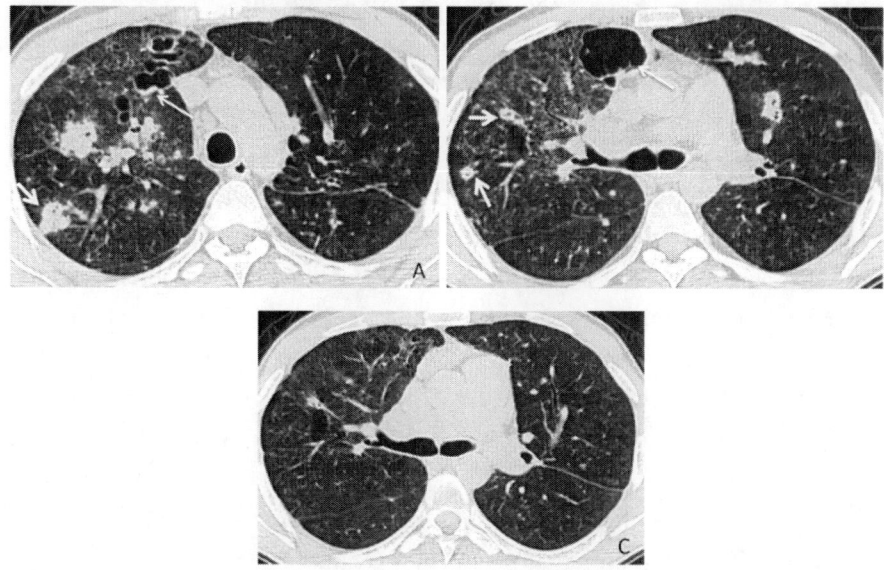

Figure 7. Pneumocystosis. Axial view with lung windowing showing excavated nodules (thick arrow) associated with pulmonary cysts (thin arrow) which resolved under treatment (C).

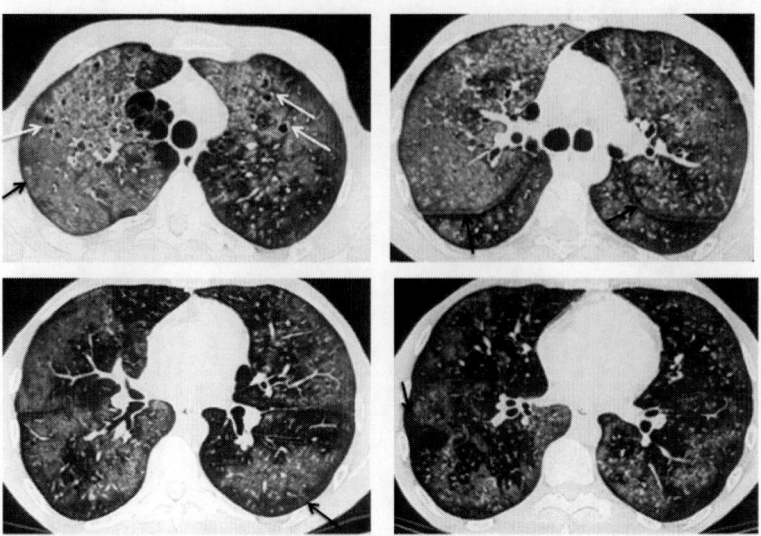

Figure 8. Pneumocystosis revealing HIV infection. Axial view with lung window. Diffuse ground glass opacities with cysts (white arrow) not affecting the peripheral cortex of the lung (black arrow). Note the upper lobe predominance.

2.1.2. Viruses and Mycoplasma Pneumoniae

Several viruses may cause AILD in adults: influenza, measles, adenovirus, herpes, varicella-zoster, cytomegalovirus (CMV), and Epstein-Barr virus. The clinical-radiological presentation of viral AILD in adults differs according to the immune status of the patient. Influenza types A and B viruses account for most viral AILD in immunocompetent adults (Franquet 2011). Immunocompromised patients are exposed mainly to CMV, herpes viruses, measles virus, and adenovirus (Kim et al. 2002). CMV is commonly found in the BAL of patients infected with HIV, but in the majority of cases it is associated with other pathogens and has no clinical impact (Lacombe et al. 2007) (Figure 9). The specific agent may be identified by tissue cultures, serologic tests, and detecting viral molecules using a polymerase chain reaction (PCR) (Franquet 2011).

Computed Tomography

Despite its limits, CT is currently the main imaging tool for assessing pulmonary viral infections. The principal elementary lesions of viral AILD are GGO with a mosaic appearance, consolidations (Figure 10), acinar nodules, a "tree-in-bud" pattern, septal thickening and bronchial wall thickening (Franquet 2011). The most frequently present pattern in viral AILD is the patchy GGO (Figure 11). CMV-induced AILD is characterized by GGO predominantly in the middle and lower regions of the lungs which may be associated with micronodules sometimes giving a miliary appearance (Allen et al. 2010, Beigelman-Aubry, Godet, and Caumes 2012, Franquet 2011) (Figure 12).

Mycoplasma Pneumoniae has the same radiological presentation as viral pneumonias.

2.1.3. Mycobacteria

Pulmonary tuberculosis may result in acute respiratory failure mainly in immunocompromised patients related to hematogenous dissemination of Koch's bacillus.

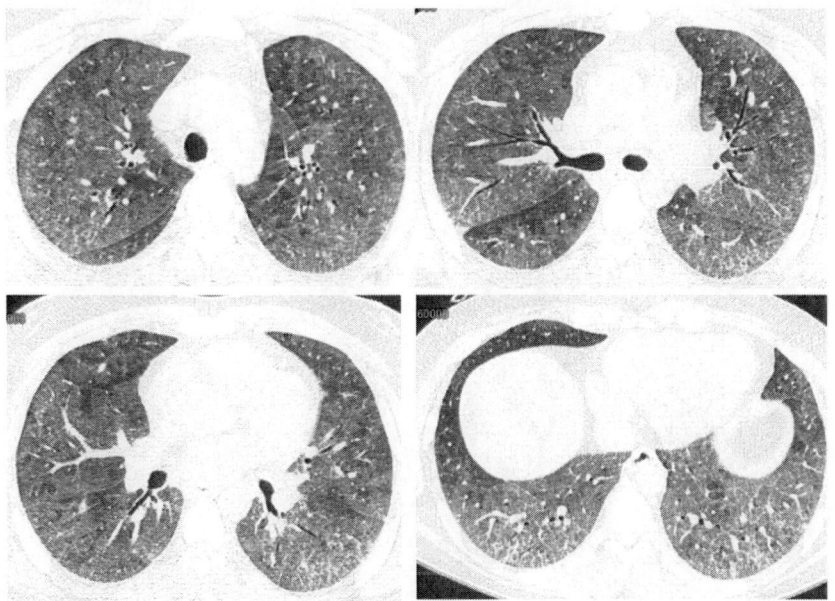

Figure 9. Axial CT scan in a human immunodeficiency virus-positive patient with *pneumocystis jiroveci* and CMV coinfection shows bilateral ground glass opacities.

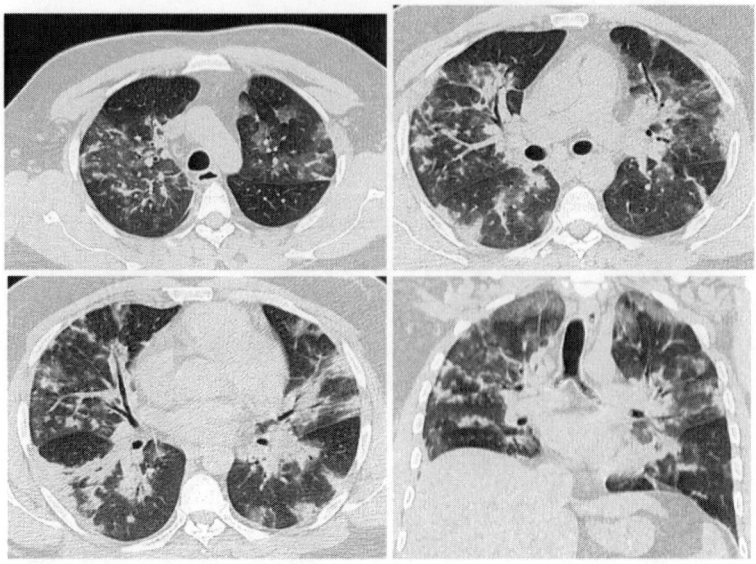

Figure 10. CT scan of a man with swine-origin influenza A (H1N1) viral infection shows bilateral peribronchovascular and peripheral areas of consolidations associated with patchy ground glass opacities.

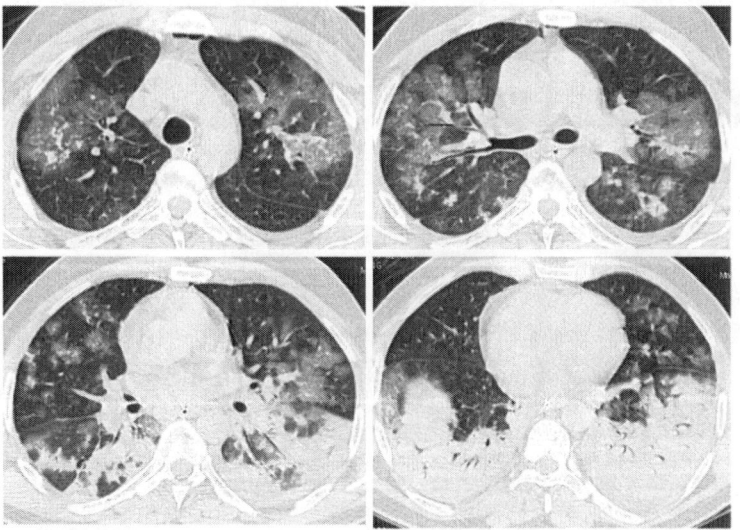

Figure 11. Axial CT scan of a patient with swine-origin influenza A (H1N1) viral infection showing bilateral patchy "ground glass" opacities associated with lower lobe consolidations.

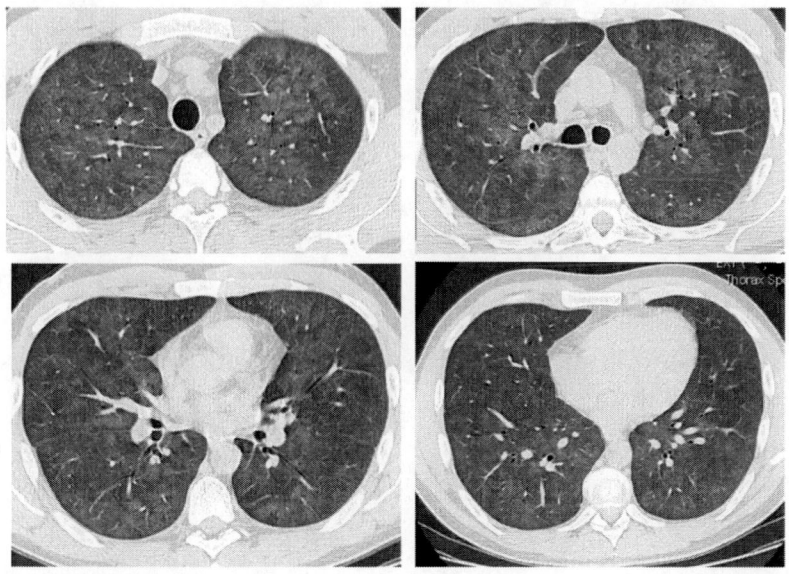

Figure 12. Axial CT scan of a 35-year-old man with CMV infection after kidney transplantation shows multiple bilateral ground glass opacities.

Atypical mycobacteria are usually non-pathogenic for humans (Griffith et al. 2007). Atypical mycobacteriosis generally occurs in immune-compromised patients. There are several germs, but the main pathogens are Mycobacterium avium, Mycobacterium Kansasii and Mycobacterium Xenopi. The most common atypical mycobacteria in HIV subjects is intracellular Mycobacterium avium complex (M. avium and M. intracellular).

Computed Tomography

Disseminated tuberculosis results in a miliary appearance in reference to innumerable small pulmonary nodules scattered randomly throughout the lungs.

In atypical mycobacteria, CT scan features are similar to that of post-primary tuberculosis. However, there are more serious rapidly progressive forms leading to AILD which are encountered in severe immunocompromised subjects, especially HIV-infected individuals. Radiologic features are nonspecific with diffuse interstitial involvement predominantly in the upper lobes associated with nodules, micronodules and consolidations (Beigelman et al. 2013). Hilar or mediastinal enlarged lymph nodes are often associated (Beigelman et al. 2013).

2.1.4. Legionellosis

The Legionellaceae are a diverse group of aerobic gram-negative bacteria. Their natural environment is in aqueous solutions or soil. Infection occurs more frequently in immunocompromised patients. Legionellosis cases are identified by urinary–antigen detection which is more sensitive than culture (Wilmes et al. 2018)

Computed Tomography

Chest CT findings include GGO and consolidation with air bronchograms. Cavitation is seen in about 10% of immunocompromised patients. Pleural effusion is often associated (Yu et al. 2010).

2.2. Pulmonary Cardiogenic Edema

Cardiogenic edema results in alveolar filling. CT scan features consist of consolidations which can be associated with bilateral GGO. These features are typically symmetrical and predominant in perihilar regions. Cardiomegaly and signs of pulmonary venous hypertension are very suggestive of the diagnosis. Pulmonary venous hypertension manifests with an enlargement of pulmonary veins with smooth septal thickening. This pattern is related to pulmonary venule enlargement along the interlobular septa (Figure 13). Bilateral pleural effusion is an additional argument for diagnosis.

At an earlier stage of interstitial edema, HR-CT features consist of regular septal thickening and peribronchovascular thickening without alveolar edema.

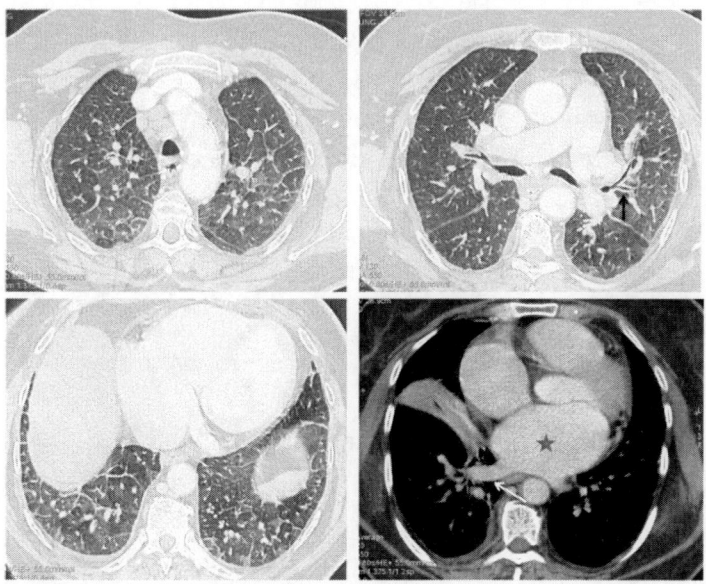

Figure 13. Axial CT showing bilateral ground glass opacity. The presence of peribronchovascular interstitial thickening (black arrow) and smooth regular interlobular septal thickening associated with pulmonary vein enlargement (white arrow) suggest hydrostatic pulmonary edema. Note heart cavity enlargement, mainly the left atrium (star).

Lesional pulmonary edema gives non-systemized bilateral diffuse or multifocal high attenuations that have a predominantly peripheral distribution at the beginning (Brauner et al. 2010). Cardiomegaly and signs of pulmonary venous hypertension are lacking.

2.3. Connective Tissue Diseases

The main connective tissue diseases accounting for AILD are polymyositis, dermatopolymyositis, systemic lupus erythematosus and mixed connective tissue disease. Three histopathological patterns can be observed during these conditions: DAD, HIA and AOP (Feuillet and Tazi 2011). AILD during inflammatory myositis is most commonly found in dermatomyositis and in the presence of antisynthetase antibodies (Feuillet and Tazi 2011).

Before confirming the diagnosis of connective tissue-related AILD, the possibility of pulmonary infection must be eliminated as it is very common in immunocompromised patients. Left heart failure could also be suggested, since cardiac involvement can be related to connective tissue diseases.

2.4. Vasculitis

Vasculitis is most often accountable for DAH, and more rarely acute eosinophilic pneumonia or DAD (Feuillet and Tazi 2011). DAH is a classic complication of vasculitis affecting small and medium-sized vessels. Granulomatosis with polyangiitis (Figures 14 and 15) and microscopic polyangiitis (Figure 16) are the most frequently encountered. DAH is less common in polyangiitis granulomatosis than in microscopic polyangiitis.

Rarely, other forms of vasculitis such as Eosinophilic Granulomatosis with Polyangiitis, Behçet's disease and rheumatoid purpura can present with AILD (Feuillet and Tazi 2011). Eosinophilic Granulomatosis with Polyangiitis is most often accountable for acute eosinophilic pneumonia (Feuillet and Tazi 2011). However, the diagnosis of hemodynamic pulmonary edema should be considered because of the specific cardiac involvement of this disease (Bernheim and McLoud 2017).

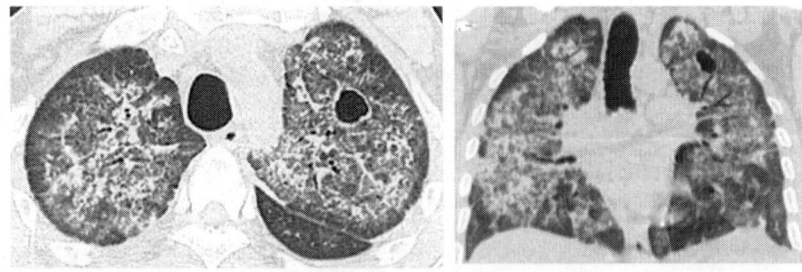

Figure 14. Diffuse alveolar hemorrhage in a 40-year-old patient with granulomatosis with polyangiitis. High-resolution CT showing central extensive "ground glass" opacities and septal thickening. Note the excavated nodule in the upper left lobe.

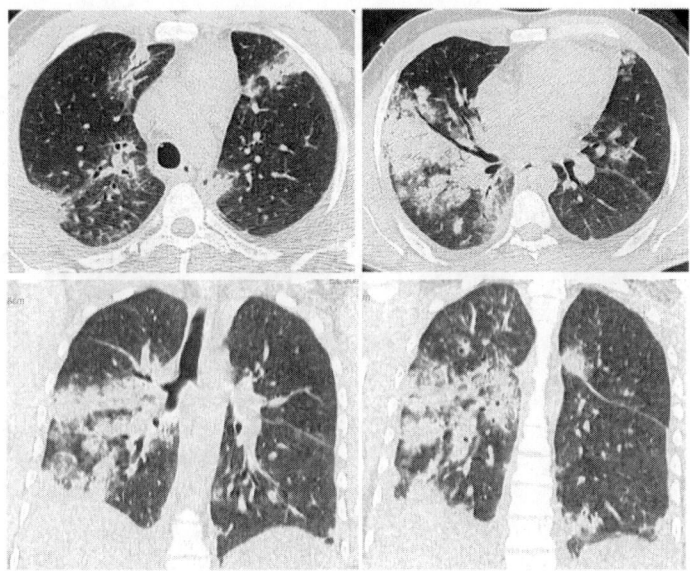

Figure 15. 23-year-old man with respiratory distress and hemoptysis. High-resolution CT scan showing multiple consolidation areas surrounded by ground glass opacities in both lungs. BAL confirmed DAH with a Golde score of 200. Positive c-ANCA was identified on immunologic tests attesting to the diagnosis of granulomatosis with polyangiitis.

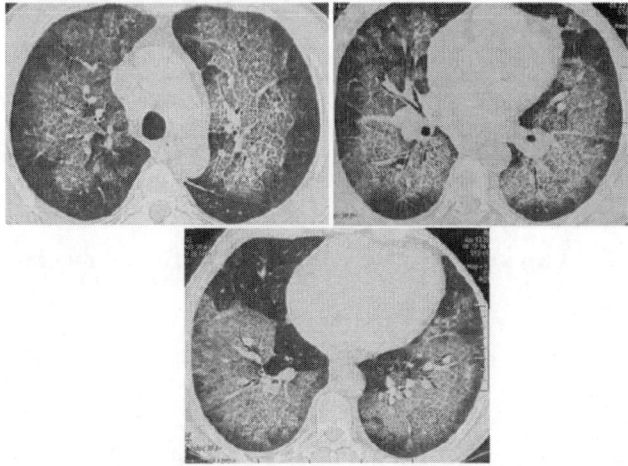

Figure 16. Diffuse alveolar hemorrhage related to microscopic polyangiitis in a 47-year-old man. Transverse CT demonstrates crazy paving appearance with central distribution.

2.5. Goodpasture Syndrome

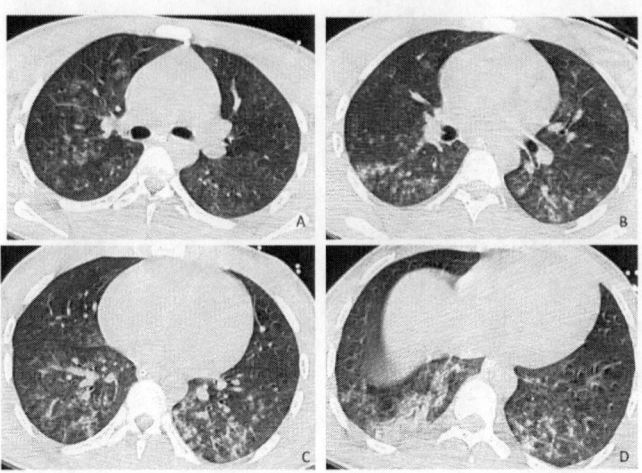

Figure 17. Goodpasture syndrome in an 18-year-old- man with hemoptysis and renal involvement. Axial CT shows subtle "ground glass opacities" in the upper lobes (A) associated with confluent centrilobular nodules surrounded by "ground glass" opacities (B and C). D image shows consolidation with air bronchograms in the right lower lobe.

Anti-glomerular basement membrane (GBM) disease, or Goodpasture syndrome, is an autoimmune disease characterized by extracapillary glomerulonephritis with linear IgG deposits along the MBG and a rapidly progressive glomerulonephritis, leading to acute renal failure. The clinical expression of the disease is mainly a pulmonary renal syndrome, associating DAH and extracapillary glomerulonephritis (Figure 17). Cases of isolated DAH, without nephropathy, have been described. The diagnosis is based on immunologic tests with a positive rate of anti-MBG antibodies present in 90% of the cases (Traclet et al. 2013).

2.6. Drugs

Drug-induced AILD results from two main mechanisms which can be associated for one single drug: direct toxicity and an immunoallergic mechanism (Mayaud et al. 2005)

There is a long list of drugs which induce AILD. This list is regularly updated in the database available on the Pneumotox website. Many nosological entities can be encountered in drug-induced AILD. Apart from DAD which is the most frequently observed, they may be acute eosinophilic pneumonia, AIAP, acute organized pneumonia or alveolar hemorrhage (Feuillet and Tazi 2011). The same drug may lead to different lesions (Mayaud et al. 2005). CT scan shows GGO, possibly associated with nodules or alveolar consolidations as well as septal thickening (Mayaud et al. 2005). The radiological appearance depends on the histological type. Propylthiouracil is known, for example, to provide ANCA-vasculitis which manifests by alveolar hemorrhage (Cordier 2006). Commonly implicated molecules are amiodarone (Figure 18), beta-blockers, statins, nitrofurantoin, phenytoin, and minocycline.

BAL has no specific results; however, it helps eliminate differential diagnoses, especially infections.

Drug imputability must be suggested relying on several arguments: chronology between drug intake and the occurrence of respiratory symptoms, literature data and the absence of another possible diagnosis. AILD being resolved once treatment is discontinued is an argument of proof (Feuillet and Tazi 2011, Mayaud et al. 2005). There are no specific histological lesions attesting to drug imputability (Mayaud et al. 2005).

Particular vigilance should be given to new drugs, including some new antineoplastics and biological therapies (anticytokines, tyrosine kinase inhibitors and so on) that are increasingly prescribed in hematological disorders or systemic diseases and which have been associated with AILD (Feuillet and Tazi 2011).

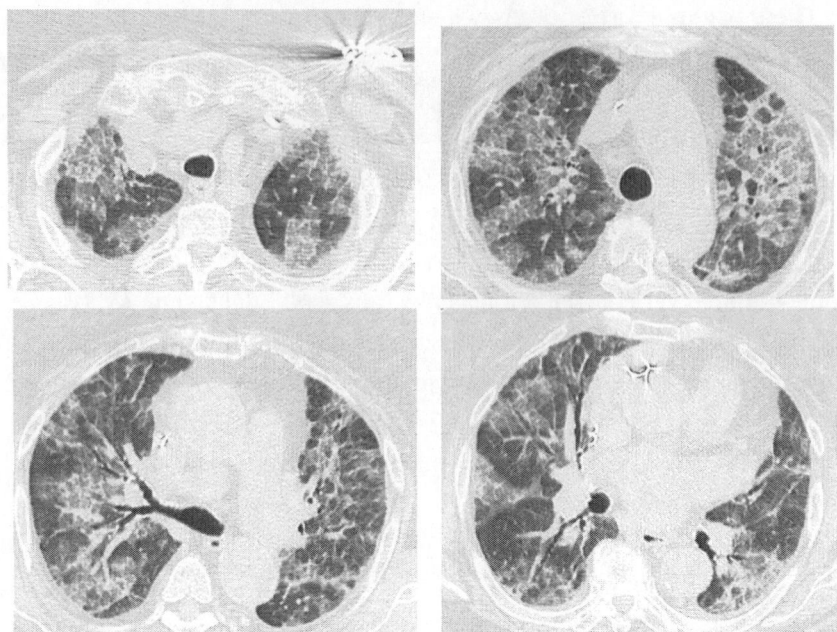

Figure 18. Chest CT of an 80-year-old-woman with respiratory distress: Bilateral diffuse ground glass opacities associated with septal thickening in relation to acute amiodarone-induced immuno-allergic pneumonia.

In addition, acute exacerbations of fibrotic interstitial lung disease have been described such as in rheumatoid arthritis patients treated with anti-TNF (Hagiwara et al. 2007). This treatment has also been associated with the potentiation of methotrexate pulmonary toxicity (Villeneuve, St-Pierre, and Haraoui 2006).

2.7. Toxics

Taking toxic drugs or inhaling them has been incriminated in AILD. Incriminated toxic substances mainly include heroin, cocaine, tobacco, fire smoke and toxic industrial vapors. Nosological contexts are DAD, AEP, DAH, and AOP. Cocaine may be responsible for pulmonary edema, HIA or acute eosinophilic pneumonia (Feuillet and Tazi 2011). A particular cocaine-related AILD named "crack lung" is due to inhalation of crack form cocaine clinically including fever, hemoptysis, hypoxemia and often respiratory failure (Restrepo et al. 2007). It corresponds to DAD associated with alveolar hemorrhage and interstitial inflammatory infiltrate rich in eosinophilic granulocytes.

Acute inhalation of fire smoke and industrial toxic fumes (dichloro, cadmium, mercury, phosgene, and so forth) may induce lesional pulmonary edema that may progress to ARDS (Rabinowitz and Siegel 2002). AOP has been described in workers exposed to textile dyes (Moya, Anto, and Taylor 1994).

Significant recent smoking may result in acute eosinophilic pneumonia (Feuillet and Tazi 2011).

2.8. Irradiation

Irradiation is a rare etiology of AILD. It occurs between 1 and 6 months after thoracic irradiation (Feuillet and Tazi 2011, Brauner et al. 2010). Its occurrence depends on the dose, its fractioning, the associated chemotherapies, and the irradiated volume (Brauner et al. 2010). It can lead to DAD with ARDS (Arpin et al. 2009). On HR-CT, it appears as consolidations or GGO typically in the irradiated fields but may overflow them. This AILD is usually cortico-sensitive, but some cases of fatal evolution have been described (Arpin et al. 2009).

A particular radiologic form of organizing pneumonia has been described, particularly in irradiated breast cancer patients (Crestani et al. 2010).

2.9. Acute Exacerbations of Fibrotic Interstitial Lung Disease

The definition and diagnostic criteria of acute exacerbation (AE) of idiopathic pulmonary fibrosis (IPF) have recently been revised. They have been defined according to the 2016 consensus as an acute clinically significant respiratory deterioration characterized by evidence of new widespread alveolar abnormalities (Collard et al. 2016). The revised diagnostic 2016 criteria include (Collard et al. 2016):

- Previous or concurrent diagnosis of idiopathic pulmonary fibrosis
- Acute worsening or development of dyspnea typically of less than one month duration
- CT with new bilateral GGO and/or consolidation superimposed on a background pattern consistent with usual interstitial pneumonia pattern
- Deterioration not fully explained by cardiac failure or fluid overload

There are risk factors that may be considered as triggers of acute exacerbation-IPF; they include cigarette smoking, baseline supplemental oxygen, gastroesophageal reflux disease, BAL, surgical lung biopsy, pulmonary resection and surgery in organs other than the lungs, and pulmonary hypertension (Spagnolo and Wuyts 2017, Papiris et al. 2014).

AE is best characterized and most common in IPF, but it may complicate a number of other fibrotic interstitial lung diseases such as nonspecific interstitial pneumonia (Figure 19), hypersensitivity pneumonia, desquamative interstitial pneumonia and asbestosis (Churg, Wright, and Tazelaar 2011).

On CT, new GGO superimposed on signs of fibrosis possibly associated with consolidation suggests AE of fibrosis (Figure 20). This diagnosis should be considered after eliminating infection or hemodynamic edema. Three variants of acute exacerbation have been described based on the distribution of GGO and consolidation on CT (Akira et al. 2008): diffuse, multifocal, and peripheral. This distinction has a prognostic impact with a fatal evolution in the cases of diffuse *pulmonary* abnormalities, a good prognosis in the case of peripheral distribution and a variable evolution in the multifocal GGO (Akira et al. 2008).

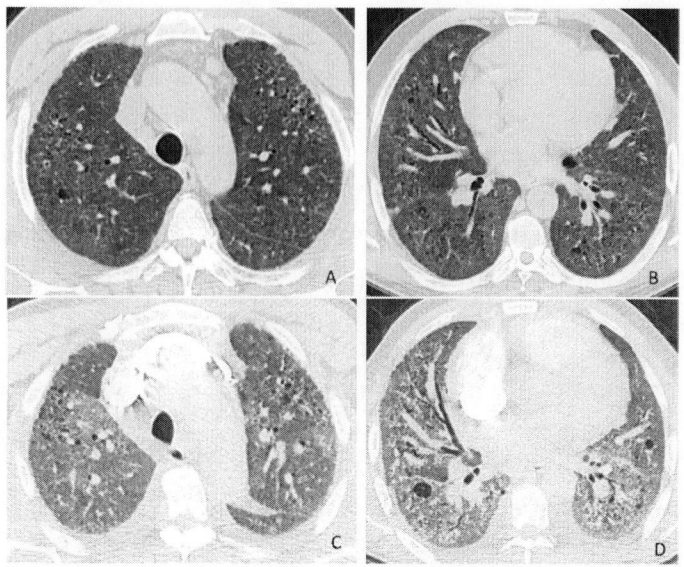

Figure 19. Computed tomography scans of a woman with nonspecific interstitial pneumonia (NSIP). A and B images show a picture of NSIP, while C and D images, taken during an acute exacerbation, show diffuse ground glass opacities superimposed on reticulation and bronchiectasis.

2.10. Acute Interstitial Pneumonia

Acute interstitial pneumonia (AIP) is a rare idiopathic interstitial pneumonia known as Hamman-Rich syndrome. It is a clinicopathologic entity characterized by rapid respiratory failure and DAD on lung biopsy (Swigris and Brown 2006, Walsh and Hansell 2010, Bonaccorsi et al. 2003).

It occurs without known cause, and the diagnosis, which is very complex, should only be suggested in the absence of an alternative explanation of the symptoms. This is a diagnosis of exclusion, and idiopathic AIP may be the first sign of connective tissue disease. In some series, antinuclear antibodies have been positive in 50% of cases (Feuillet and Tazi 2011). It has been proposed that infectious agents or toxins could trigger the process (Martinez-Risquez et al. 2018, Bonaccorsi et al. 2003).

On HRCT scan, there are symmetric diffuse GGO with a patchy consolidation usually predominant in gravity dependent areas (Bonaccorsi et al. 2003) (Figure 21). Interlobular septal and bronchovascular bundle thickening, intralobular reticular opacities as well as pleural effusions have also been reported (Swigris and Brown 2006). Traction bronchiectasis and bronchiolectasis are present in the proliferative phase of DAD (Swigris and Brown 2006, Ichikado 2014). Honeycombing may develop later in the course of the disease (Ichikado 2014).

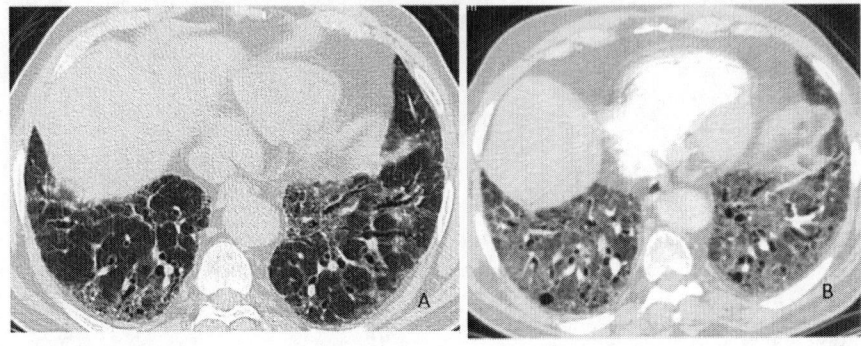

Figure 20. Illustrative example of high-resolution CT of idiopathic pulmonary fibrosis at baseline (A) and with acute exacerbation (B).

A differential diagnosis of AIP is acute respiratory distress syndrome (ARDS) which has the same radiologic and pathologic pattern but is not idiopathic (Bonaccorsi et al. 2003). Parenchymal abnormalities in AIP are predominant in the lower lung zone and have a bilateral symmetric distribution with a higher frequency of honeycombing compared to ARDS (Ichikado 2014).

High-resolution computed tomography scan. Bilateral areas of alveolar filling are evident in the gravitational areas of the lungs.

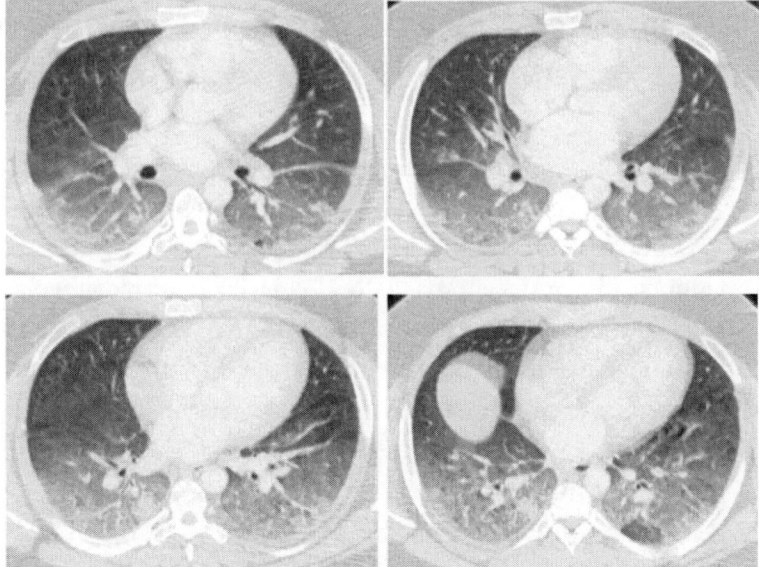

Figure 21. Exsudative phase of the Hamman Rich syndrome.

2.11. Rare Etiologies

Some rare causes should be known (Feuillet and Tazi 2011):

- Tumoral causes (lymphoma, carcinoma) can lead to acute pulmonary tumor infiltration in the form of lymphangitic carcinomatosis.
- Pulmonary leukostasis in the context of acute leukemias has been described and should be considered in this particular context after eliminating other causes such as infection, hemorrhaging and so on
- Exceptional cases of acute forms of sarcoidosis have been reported.
- Pulmonary and hematopoietic stem cell transplants (autologous or allogeneic) are also rare causes of AILD with DAD.
- Acute thoracic syndrome complicating sickle cell disease.

3. Practical Diagnostic Approach in Imaging of Acute Infiltrative Lung Disease

AILDs are relatively common conditions in patients admitted to intensive care units. They include various etiologies that have clinical and radiological similarity. The clinician and radiologist should collaborate to achieve a rational diagnostic approach. Reasoning based on the predominant pattern and lesion distribution on the CT scan can help suggest the diagnosis. CT-scan interpretation should be integrated within the clinical context and BAL data. The non-specific character of radiological images accounts for CT-scan limitations. CT scans should be prescribed as soon as possible before undergoing BAL. In fact, this procedure may distort radiological features. CT-scan is useful for guiding the site of the BAL. In addition, radiological outcome may worsen with extension consolidations masking the elementary lesions of the AILD. It would always be interesting, in these cases, to analyze the areas where lesions are less pronounced to look for a hidden pattern. A diagnostic AILD approach should be stereotyped based on answering clear and hierarchical questions:

(a) First, Am I Facing Left Heart Failure?

This diagnosis is relatively easy to consider on imaging.

(b) Is It an Infection?

In general, the clinico-biological data are suggestive including fever associated with a biological inflammatory syndrome. However, an isolated fever must be considered with reserve since it may be associated, for example, with systemic diseases, acute eosinophilic pneumonia, drug-induced pneumonitis and hypersensitivity pneumonia. Likewise, the biological inflammatory syndrome may be lacking in some patients or with some germs.

Two groups should be distinguished: immunocompetent patients in whom virus induced-AILD especially influenza viruses are the most common etiology; and immunocompromised patients, in whom P. jirovecii, CMV, or mycoplasma must be suggested.

A diagnosis of pneumocystosis is relatively simple in the case of typical radiological features. The diagnosis should be suggested in immunocompromised patients with AILD mainly made up of GGO and should be confirmed by the BAL.

CMV induced-pneumonia is to be considered in particular cases, including hematopoietic organ and stem cell transplant recipients and HIV-infected patients with a CD4 count of less than 100 (Franquet 2011).

Finally, in the presence of DAH on a CT scan with the classic "crazy paving" pattern, the diagnosis of leptospirosis should be considered.

In summary, in infection induced-AILD, CT scans can help suggest the diagnosis, especially in typical cases, but confirmation is essentially based on bacteriological and immunological examinations.

(c) In the Absence of Pulmonary Edema and Infection, Which Diagnoses can be Considered?

In this situation, the CT scan is limited, with nonspecific radiological appearance of non-infectious and non-cardiogenic AILD. Etiologies are numerous, dominated by drugs, vasculitis, connective tissue diseases, and tumors. The diagnosis is based on a combination of clinical, biological, radiological, cytological (BAL) and rarely pathological sample (obtained by surgical lung biopsies) arguments.

A clinical examination with careful history-taking is very helpful in highlighting predisposing factors, drug intake and extra respiratory signs, especially cutaneous ones that would point towards a systemic disease or a drug cause. Hemoptysis indicates a DAH mainly related to vasculitis.

Biological tests may detect associated renal involvement and would point to a pulmonary-renal syndrome most often related to vasculitis or

Goodpasture syndrome. Immunologic tests may also help point to a systemic disease.

Chest CT scan features are mainly GGO more or less associated with consolidations and a reticular pattern. It can guide the BAL site and help suggest a diagnosis in a number of cases by pointing to a particular nosological context:

- DAH which can be suggested in the presence of a diffuse "crazy paving" pattern sparing the subpleural regions associated with hemoptysis.
- AIAP: in front of a AILD made up mainly of GGO predominant in the lower lobes.
- Acute organized pneumonia with peribronchovascular and peripheral consolidations which may be surrounded by GGO leading to the halo sign.

Clinical, biological, cytological and radiological data lead to the diagnosis in most cases. Thus, predominant eosinophils cells on BAL (more than 25%) in the presence of AILD made up of consolidations and GGO leads to an AEP diagnosis. DAH suggested by a CT scan and confirmed by BAL in the presence of pANCA indicates the diagnosis of a microscopic polyangiitis. In the presence of cANCA, the diagnosis of garnulomatosis with polyangiitis disease can be made.

In case of any drug intake, the website Pneumotox would be of great help for the diagnosis.

Finally, when the exhaustive etiological investigation is negative and in the presence of AILD made up of bilateral and symmetrical consolidations and GGO predominant in the lower lobes of the lungs, the diagnosis of AIP should be considered.

CONCLUSION

AILD is a heterogeneous group of lung disorders resulting from several causes. A CT scan, even with its nonspecific character, remains a useful examination in diagnosis. A positive diagnosis is based on integrating clinical, biological, cytological and imaging arguments.

REFERENCES

Akira, M., Kozuka, T., Yamamoto, S. & Sakatani, M. (2008). "Computed tomography findings in acute exacerbation of idiopathic pulmonary fibrosis." *Am J Respir Crit Care Med*, *178* (4), 372-8. doi: 10.1164/rccm.200709-1365OC.

Allen, C. M., Al-Jahdali, H. H., Irion, K. L., Al Ghanem, S., Gouda, A. & Khan, A. N. (2010). "Imaging lung manifestations of HIV/AIDS." *Ann Thorac Med*, *5* (4), 201-16. doi: 10.4103/1817-1737.69106.

Allen, J. (2006). "Acute eosinophilic pneumonia." *Semin Respir Crit Care Med*, *27* (2), 142-7. doi: 10.1055/s-2006-939517.

Arpin, D., Mahe, M. A., Servois, V. & Claude, L. (2009). "[Predictive factors for acute radiation pneumonitis]." *Rev Pneumol Clin*, *65* (3), 177-86. doi: 10.1016/j.pneumo.2009.03.011.

Beigelman-Aubry, C., Godet, C. & Caumes, E. (2012). "Lung infections: the radiologist's perspective." *Diagn Interv Imaging*, *93* (6), 431-40. doi: 10.1016/j.diii.2012.04.021.

Beigelman, C., Brauner, M., Soussan, M., Arrigoni, P. P. & Brillet, P. Y. (2013). "PATHOLOGIE INFECTIEUSE." In *Imagerie Thoracique de l'adulte et de l'enfant*, edited by C. Baunin, C. Beigelman, M. Brauner, M. F. Carette, M. P. Debray, H. Ducou le Pointe, C. Durand, G. Durand, M. El Hajjam, P. Fajadet, G. Ferretti, P. A. Gevenois, B. Ghaye, J. Giron, M. Hackx, D. Jeanbourquin, A. Khalil, P. Lacombe, A. Lacout, A. Madani, S. Maître, C. Meunier, L. Metge, B. Padovani, A. Resten, P. Scillia and D. Tack, 513-583.

Bernheim, A. & McLoud, T. (2017). "A Review of Clinical and Imaging Findings in Eosinophilic Lung Diseases." *AJR Am J Roentgenol*, *208* (5), 1002-1010. doi: 10.2214/AJR.16.17315.

Bonaccorsi, A., Cancellieri, A., Chilosi, M., Trisolini, R., Boaron, M., Crimi, N. & Poletti, V. (2003). "Acute interstitial pneumonia: report of a series." *Eur Respir J*, *21* (1), 187-91.

Brauner, M., Ben Romdhane, H., Brillet, P. Y., Freynet, O., Dion, G. & Valeyre, D. (2010). "[Imaging findings in intersitial lung diseases]." *Presse Med*, *39* (1), 73-84. doi: 10.1016/j.lpm.2009.09.014.

Churg, A., Wright, J. L. & Tazelaar, H. D. (2011). "Acute exacerbations of fibrotic interstitial lung disease." *Histopathology*, *58* (4), 525-30. doi: 10.1111/j.1365-2559.2010.03650.x.

Collard, H. R., Ryerson, C. J., Corte, T. J., Jenkins, G., Kondoh, Y., Lederer, D. J., Lee, J. S., Maher, T. M., Wells, A. U., Antoniou, K. M., Behr, J., Brown, K. K., Cottin, V., Flaherty, K. R., Fukuoka, J., Hansell, D. M., Johkoh, T., Kaminski, N., Kim, D. S., Kolb, M., Lynch, D. A., Myers, J. L., Raghu, G., Richeldi, L., Taniguchi, H. & Martinez, F. J. (2016). "Acute Exacerbation of Idiopathic Pulmonary Fibrosis. An International Working Group Report." *Am J Respir Crit Care Med*, *194* (3), 265-75. doi: 10.1164/rccm.201604-0801CI.

Collard, H. R. & Schwarz, M. I. (2004). "Diffuse alveolar hemorrhage." *Clin Chest Med*, *25* (3), 583-92, vii. doi: 10.1016/j.ccm.2004.04.007.

Cordier, J. F. (2006). "[Diffuse alveolar hemorrhage: when anyone thinks? Which balance?]." *Rev Mal Respir*, *23* (6), 749-50.

Crestani, B., Taille, C., Borie, R., Debray, M. P., Danel, C., Dombret, M. C. & Aubier, M. (2010). "[Organizing pneumonia]." *Presse Med*, *39* (1), 126-33. doi: 10.1016/j.lpm.2009.10.007.

Daimon, T., Johkoh, T., Sumikawa, H., Honda, O., Fujimoto, K., Koga, T., Arakawa, H., Yanagawa, M., Inoue, A., Mihara, N., Tomiyama, N., Nakamura, H. & Sugiyama, Y. (2008). "Acute eosinophilic pneumonia: Thin-section CT findings in 29 patients." *Eur J Radiol*, *65* (3), 462-7. doi: 10.1016/j.ejrad.2007.04.012.

De Giacomi, F., Vassallo, R., Yi, E. S. & Ryu, J. H. (2018). "Acute Eosinophilic Pneumonia. Causes, Diagnosis, and Management." *Am J Respir Crit Care Med*, *197* (6), 728-736. doi: 10.1164/rccm.201710-1967CI.

Feuillet, S. & Tazi, A. (2011). "[Acute interstitial pneumonia: diagnostic approach and management]." *Rev Mal Respir*, *28* (6), 809-22. doi: 10.1016/j.rmr.2011.01.010.

Franks, T. J. & Galvin, J. R. (2010). "Hypersensitivity Pneumonitis: Essential Radiologic and Pathologic Findings." *Surg Pathol Clin*, *3* (1), 187-98. doi: 10.1016/j.path.2010.03.005.

Franquet, T. (2011). "Imaging of pulmonary viral pneumonia." *Radiology*, *260* (1), 18-39. doi: 10.1148/radiol.11092149.

Griffith, D. E., Aksamit, T., Brown-Elliott, B. A., Catanzaro, A., Daley, C., Gordin, F., Holland, S. M., Horsburgh, R., Huitt, G., Iademarco, M. F., Iseman, M., Olivier, K., Ruoss, S., von Reyn, C. F., Wallace, R. J., Jr. Winthrop, K. & A. T. S. Mycobacterial Diseases Subcommittee, Society American Thoracic, and America Infectious Disease Society of. (2007). "An official ATS/IDSA statement: diagnosis, treatment, and prevention of nontuberculous mycobacterial diseases." *Am J Respir Crit Care Med*, *175* (4), 367-416. doi: 10.1164/rccm.200604-571ST.

Hagiwara, K., Sato, T., Takagi-Kobayashi, S., Hasegawa, S., Shigihara, N. & Akiyama, O. (2007). "Acute exacerbation of preexisting interstitial lung disease after administration of etanercept for rheumatoid arthritis." *J Rheumatol*, *34* (5), 1151-4.

Ichikado, K. (2014). "High-resolution computed tomography findings of acute respiratory distress syndrome, acute interstitial pneumonia, and acute exacerbation of idiopathic pulmonary fibrosis." *Semin Ultrasound CT MR*, *35* (1), 39-46. doi: 10.1053/j.sult.2013.10.007.

Kim, E. A., Lee, K. S., Primack, S. L., Yoon, H. K., Byun, H. S., Kim, T. S., Suh, G. Y., Kwon, O. J. & Han, J. (2002). "Viral pneumonias in adults: radiologic and pathologic findings." *Radiographics*, *22*, Spec No: S137-49. doi: 10.1148/radiographics.22.suppl_1.g02oc15s137.

Knutsen, A. P., Temprano, J., Bhatla, D. & Slavin, R. G. (2019). "Hypersensitivity Pneumonitis and Eosinophilic Lung Diseases." In *Kendig's Disorders of the Respiratory Tract in Children*, edited by R. Wilmott, A. Bush, R. Deterding and F. Ratjen, 944-967.

Lacombe, C., Lewin, M., Monnier-Cholley, L., Pacanowski, J., Poirot, J. L., Arrive, L. & Tubiana, J. M. (2007). "[Imaging of thoracic pathology in patients with AIDS]." *J Radiol*, *88* (9 Pt 1), 1145-54.

Marchiori, E., Muller, N. L., Soares Souza, A., Jr. Escuissato, D. L., Gasparetto, E. L. & Franquet, T. (2005). "Pulmonary disease in patients with AIDS: high-resolution CT and pathologic findings." *AJR Am J Roentgenol*, *184* (3), 757-64. doi: 10.2214/ajr.184.3.01840757.

Martinez-Risquez, M. T., Friaza, V., de la Horra, C., Martin-Juan, J., Calderon, E. J. & Medrano, F. J. (2018). "Pneumocystis jirovecii infection in patients with acute interstitial pneumonia." *Rev Clin Esp*, *218* (8), 417-420. doi: 10.1016/j.rce.2018.04.016.

Mayaud, C., Fartoukh, M., Parrot, A., Cadranel, J., Milleron, B. & Akoun, G. (2005). "[Drug-associated interstitial lung disease: a diagnostic challenge]." *Rev Pneumol Clin*, *61* (3), 179-85.

Moya, C., Anto, J. M. & Taylor, A. J. (1994). "Outbreak of organising pneumonia in textile printing sprayers. Collaborative Group for the Study of Toxicity in Textile Aerographic Factories." *Lancet*, *344* (8921), 498-502.

Papiris, S. A., Kagouridis, K., Kolilekas, L., Bouros, D. & Manali, E. D. (2014). "Idiopathic pulmonary fibrosis acute exacerbations: where are we now?" *Expert Rev Respir Med*, *8* (3), 271-3. doi: 10.1586/17476348.2014.896206.

Parambil, J. G., Myers, J. L., Aubry, M. C. & Ryu, J. H. (2007). "Causes and prognosis of diffuse alveolar damage diagnosed on surgical lung biopsy." *Chest*, *132* (1), 50-7. doi: 10.1378/chest.07-0104.

Rabinowitz, P. M. & Siegel, M. D. (2002). "Acute inhalation injury." *Clin Chest Med*, *23* (4), 707-15.

Restrepo, C. S., Carrillo, J. A., Martinez, S., Ojeda, P., Rivera, A. L. & Hatta, A. (2007). "Pulmonary complications from cocaine and cocaine-based substances: imaging manifestations." *Radiographics*, *27* (4), 941-56. doi: 10.1148/rg.274065144.

Spagnolo, P. & Wuyts, W. (2017). "Acute exacerbations of interstitial lung disease: lessons from idiopathic pulmonary fibrosis." *Curr Opin Pulm Med*, *23* (5), 411-417. doi: 10.1097/MCP.0000000000000405.

Swigris, J. J. & Brown, K. K. (2006). "Acute interstitial pneumonia and acute exacerbations of idiopathic pulmonary fibrosis." *Semin Respir Crit Care Med*, *27* (6), 659-67. doi: 10.1055/s-2006-957337.

Traclet, J., Lazor, R., Cordier, J. F. & Cottin, V. (2013). "[Alveolar hemorrhage]." *Rev Med Interne*, *34* (4), 214-23. doi: 10.1016/j.revmed.2012.08.002.

Villeneuve, E., St-Pierre, A. & Haraoui, B. (2006). "Interstitial pneumonitis associated with infliximab therapy." *J Rheumatol*, *33* (6), 1189-93.

Walsh, S. L. & Hansell, D. M. (2010). "Diffuse interstitial lung disease: overlaps and uncertainties." *Eur Radiol*, *20* (8), 1859-67. doi: 10.1007/s00330-010-1737-3.

Wilmes, D., Coche, E., Rodriguez-Villalobos, H. & Kanaan, N. (2018). "Bacterial pneumonia in kidney transplant recipients." *Respir Med*, *137*, 89-94. doi: 10.1016/j.rmed.2018.02.022.

Yu, H., Higa, F., Hibiya, K., Furugen, M., Sato, Y., Shinzato, T., Haranaga, S., Yara, S., Tateyama, M., Fujita, J. & Li, H. (2010). "Computed tomographic features of 23 sporadic cases with Legionella pneumophila pneumonia." *Eur J Radiol*, *74* (3), e73-8. doi: 10.1016/j.ejrad.2009.04.011.

In: Interstitial Lung Disease ISBN: 978-1-53616-246-2
Editor: Liva T. Villadsen © 2019 Nova Science Publishers, Inc.

Chapter 3

IMAGING OF IDIOPATHIC AND CONNECTIVITIS-ASSOCIATED INTERSTITIAL PNEUMONIAS

Monia Attia[1], MD, Mariem Affes[1], Henda Nèji[1], MD, Houda Gharsalli[2], MD, Ines Baccouche[1], MD, Khaoula Ben Miled-M'rad[1], MD and Saoussen Hantous-Zannad[1], MD

[1]Imaging Department,
[2]"D"Pulmonology Department
Abderrahmen Mami Hospital, Ariana, Tunisia
Faculty of Medicine of Tunis, Tunis El Manar University,
Tunis, Tunisia

ABSTRACT

Interstitial pneumonias are a group of heterogeneous lung diseases that may be idiopathic or associated with an underlying abnormality such as connectivitis.

Imaging plays an essential role in characterizing this group of disorders and can often help identify the diagnosis.

A chest X-ray is often the first examination to suggest lung interstitial involvement.

However, it provides only limited information and is primarily used to rule out a differential diagnosis, such as left heart failure.

High-resolution computed tomography (HRCT) is more sensitive and accurate in diagnosing interstitial lung disease.

It plays a central role in recognizing and classifying this group of diseases through specific CT features and patterns which are highly suggestive of a subtype of interstitial pneumonia.

However, many of them share common imaging characteristics with significant overlap.

HRCT aims to find associated signs which may lead to suspicions of an associated connective tissue disease. It also allows a patient's prognosis to be evaluated and followed up with.

Although HR-CT is a cornerstone of an interstitial pneumonia diagnosis, a multidisciplinary approach is mandatory to best manage the patient.

1. INTRODUCTION

Interstitial pneumonias include a group of diffuse parenchymal lung diseases with a variety of clinicopathologic presentations.

They may be idiopathic or associated to various conditions, especially connective tissue diseases [1].

Idiopathic interstitial lung pneumonias (IIPs) were first classified internationally in 2002 by the American Thoracic Society/European Respiratory Society International Multidisciplinary Consensus classification. This new classification defined a set of histologic patterns that provided the basis for a final clinico–radiologic–pathologic diagnosis [2].

An update in 2013 included an additional classification based on disease behavior. In fact, IIPs are a heterogeneous group of diseases with various prognoses and responses to treatment [3].

In 2018, a new revision of the ATS/ERS classification was published dividing IIPs into chronic fibrosing IIPs (idiopathic pulmonary fibrosis (IPF) and idiopathic nonspecific interstitial pneumonia (NSIP)); smoking-related

IIPs; acute or subacute IIPs (cryptogenic organizing pneumonia (COP) and acute interstitial pneumonia); and rare IIPs (lymphoid interstitial pneumonia and idiopathic pleuroparenchymal fibroelastosis) [3, 4].

2. Idiopathic Pulmonary Fibrosis

IPF is a chronic progressive fibrosing lung disease of unknown cause characterized by the histopathologic pattern of usual interstitial pneumonia (UIP) [5].

Although UIP patterns are frequently seen in patients suffering from IPF, they may also develop in association with drug and dust exposure, chronic hypersensitivity pneumonitis, connective tissue diseases, and asbestos exposure. These secondary causes should be excluded before classifying UIP as idiopathic and thus the interstitial pneumonia as IPF [1].

2.1. Histologic Findings

The UIP histological pattern is characterized by a spatial and temporal heterogeneity.

A lung biopsy shows a combination of interstitial inflammation, fibroblastic foci, fibrosis, and honeycombing alternating with normal regions of lung within the same lung biopsic sample [6].

2.2. HRCT Patterns

The CT findings of UIP pointing to the heterogeneous fibrosing process vary.

HRCT features frequently seen in UIP include honeycombing, bronchiectasis and bronchiolectasis traction, fine reticulation and, less frequently, ground-glass opacities [1].

The official ATS/ERS/JRS/ALAT Clinical Practice Guideline published in September 2018 advocates for the use of four recent categories which incorporate HRCT features to diagnose UIP. These categories include a "UIP pattern," "probable UIP pattern," "indeterminate UIP pattern" and "alternative diagnosis" [4, 7].

2.2.1. UIP Pattern

Honeycombing is the hallmark radiologic pattern of UIP that must be present for a definite diagnosis of UIP. It is often seen in association with reticulations, broncho vascular distortion and bronchiolectasis.

The typical distribution of UIP is bilateral and symmetric with a craniocaudal gradient.

Subpleural regions are predominately concerned.

An asymmetric or diffuse disease involving both upper and lower lobes is rare but may occur.

Surgical lung biopsy is not required for the final diagnosis of UIP according to the latest guidelines. In fact, this UIP pattern on HRCT has a positive predictive value of about 90% in a definitive pathological UIP diagnosis [4, 7].

Ground glass opacities (GGO) may be present, but they are not a dominant feature and are usually accompanied by a superimposed reticular pattern [4].

When analyzing CT images of a UIP pattern, radiologists should carefully consider every nodule and parenchymal mass, especially in areas of fibrosis. UIP is indeed a risk factor of lung cancer with an incidence of about 10–15%, usually occurring in the lower lobes [1].

Probable UIP is considered when HRCT images show subpleural, basal-predominant reticular abnormalities with peripheral traction bronchiectasis or bronchiolectasis without honeycombing lesions. Ground glass opacities may be present in probable UIP, but they are not a dominant feature.

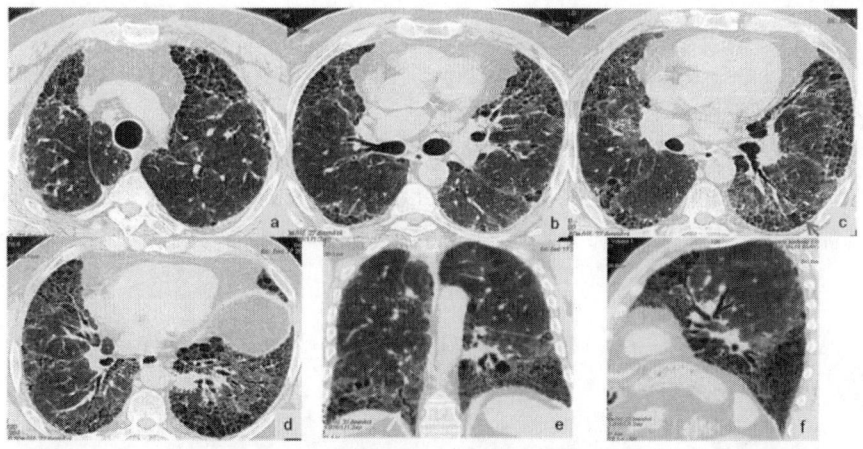

Figure 1. Usual interstitial pneumonia (UIP) pattern: axial (a,b,c,d) coronal (e) and sagittal (f) reconstructions showing peripheral honeycombing lesions (blue arrow), predominate in lower lobes, accompanied by traction bronchiectasis (yellow arrow) and scattered peripheral reticular opacities. Honeycombing is the dominant feature, typical for a UIP pattern. Neoplastic nodule in the left lower lobe (red arrow).

2.2.2. Probable UIP Pattern

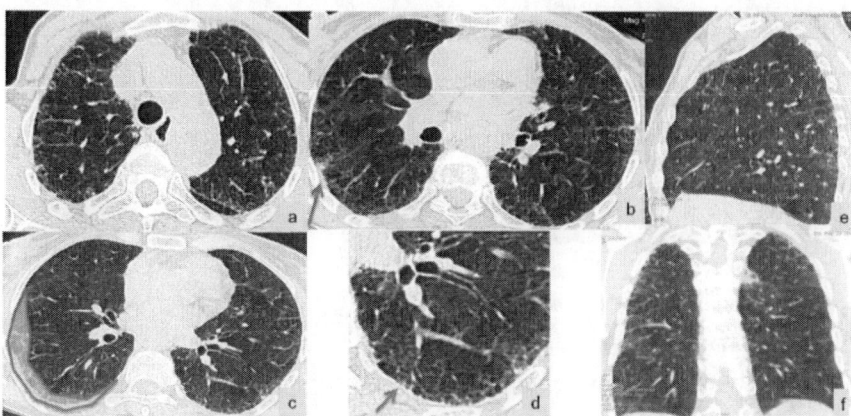

Figure 2. Probable UIP pattern. (a–c) Transverse computed tomography sections. (d) magnified axial view of the left lower lobe. (e, f) sagittal and coronal reconstructions illustrating the presence of a reticular pattern with peripheral bronchiolectasis (blue arrow). It predominates in the subpleural and basal regions. Mild ground glass opacities in the subpleural areas (red arrow) and the absence of honeycombing.

2.2.3. Indeterminate UIP Pattern

This category should be considered when a radiological pattern meets neither the typical UIP nor the probable UIP pattern.

On HRCT images, there is subtle reticulation or distortion associated with mild GGO ("early UIP pattern") with a subpleural basal distribution.

A prone inspiratory acquisition should be performed in order to rule out gravity dependent atelectasis.

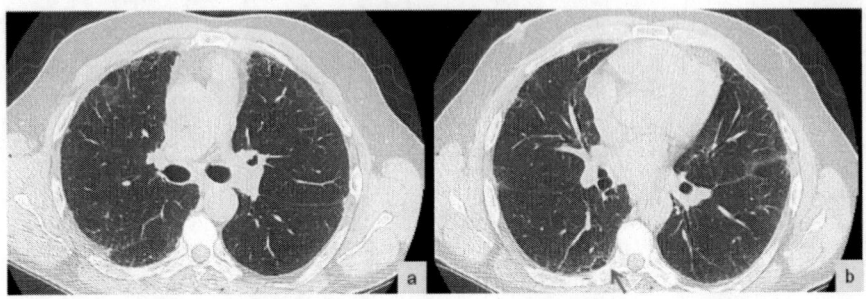

Figure 3. Indeterminate usual interstitial pneumonia (UIP) pattern (early UIP pattern). (a and b) Transverse computed tomography images showing ground glass opacities and subtle reticulation in the subpleural areas (blue arrow) with a mild basal predominance.

2.2.4. Alternative Diagnosis

In some cases of fibrotic lung disease, IPF is suspected clinically but the HRCT pattern matches an alternative diagnosis such as a cyst, mosaic attenuation, predominant GGO, micronodules, nodules or consolidation.

Except when the radiological features present a peribronchovascular, perilymphatic distribution or upper or mid-lung predominance, the diagnosis of UIP should be reconsidered.

Other signs may also suggest an alternate diagnosis rather than IPF, such as pleural plaques (asbestosis), effusion (CTD, drugs), a dilated esophagus (CTD), or extensive lymph node enlargement [4].

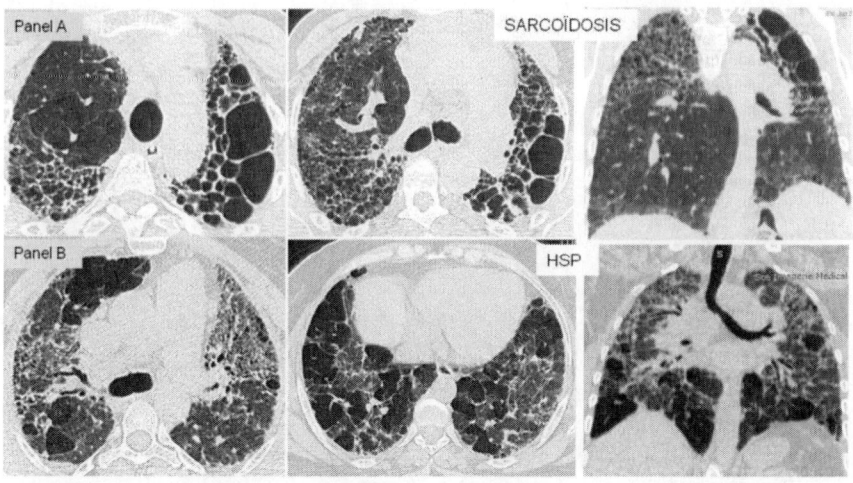

Figure 4. Computed tomography (CT) pattern suggestive of an alternative diagnosis for lung fibrosis. Panel A reveals predominant upper lobe fibrosis similar to fibrosing sarcoidosis, (Panel B) Transverse CT sections showing a heterogeneous pattern of ILP, sparing some secondary pulmonary lobules in lung bases suggests chronic hypersensitivity pneumonitis.

2.3. Acute Exacerbation

Rapidly progressive shortness of breath in a patient followed for IPF is usually caused by a pulmonary infection, pulmonary embolism, pneumothorax or congestive heart failure.

However, in some cases, no etiology is found.

These patients are diagnosed as having acute exacerbation or accelerated deterioration of IPF.

The characteristic high-resolution CT findings of acute exacerbation of IPF consist of bilateral ground glass opacities and areas of consolidation superimposed on a background of reticulation and honeycombing.

These ground glass opacities are of recent appearance concomitant to the clinical signs. They are located in the areas of honeycombing lesions.

The most common histologic pattern of acute lung injury is diffuse alveolar damage. Less commonly, patients may have organizing pneumonia or extensive fibroblastic foci, both of which are a better prognosis [8].

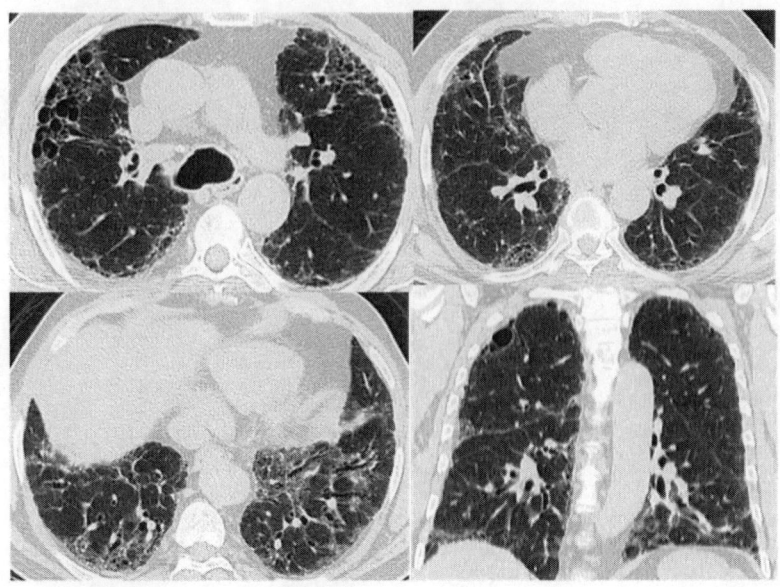

Figure 5. a. UIP pattern in a 76-year-old man followed for 5 years. b. Same patient 2 years later consulting for recent breath shortness: acute exacerbation of the IPF: UIP pattern associated with ground glass opacities without any etiology found in clinical investigations.

2.4. UIP Pattern Associated with CTD

Although a UIP pattern is usually seen in IPF, it may be the radiological pattern of lung interstitial pneumonia associated with connective tissue disease.

In fact, a UIP pattern is the most common interstitial pneumonia seen in rheumatoid arthritis (RA) [9].

IPF has a poor prognosis with median survival time ranging from 2.5–3.5 years after diagnosis [1].

Nevertheless, some authors reported a better prognosis in CTD associated UIP because of fewer fibroblastic foci, less microscopic honeycombing, and more lymphoid aggregates with germinal centers in a histopathological study [10].

That may also be due to the younger age of patients having CTD as well as their better baseline pulmonary function [10, 11].

Concerning radiological findings, HRCT features are similar in UIP associated with IPF or CTD [12].

However, a recent study tried to rule out three CT signs in order to differentiate between UIP associated with CTD-ILD and UIP associated with IPF.

These signs are fibrosis features in the anterior region of the superior lobes in association with lower lobe involvement (the "anterior upper lobe" sign); exuberant honeycomb-like cysts making up 70% of fibrotic lung portions (the "exuberant honeycombing" sign); and marked fibrosis in lung bases with sharp demarcation in the craniocaudal plane without lateral extension on coronal images (the "straight-edge" sign) [13].

3. NON-SPECIFIC INTERSTITIAL PNEUMONIA (NSIP)

NSIP was first described in 1994 as a distinct form of interstitial lung disease characterized by homogeneous alveolar wall thickening caused by inflammation or fibrosis [2].

NSIP is most often associated with underlying connective tissue disease but can also occur in an idiopathic form [14].

3.1. Histologic Subtypes

There are three subtypes of NSIP: cellular, mixed and fibrotic patterns.

Cellular NSIP is characterized by a high level of interstitial inflammation associated with little fibrosis.

In contrast, fibrosing NSIP predominately consists of a fibrosing interstitial infiltration which usually preserves the alveolar architecture [15, 16].

The histologic hallmark of NSIP is its temporal and spatial homogeneity. On a lung biopsy, all lesions are approximately the same age and in the same stage, unlike in UIP histologic patterns [1, 6].

3.2. HRCT Patterns

Two features mainly characterize NSIP: ground glass opacities and reticulations.

In cellular NSIP, ground glass opacity is the dominant CT finding corresponding histologically to homogeneous interstitial inflammation.

CT markers of fibrosis are found in various proportions, including reticulations, traction bronchiectasis, and lower lobe volume loss.

Honeycombing is not a predominant feature of NSIP and tends to be mild when present, occurring almost exclusively in patients with fibrotic NSIP [17].

NSIP usually has a bilateral symmetric distribution with lower lobe predominance.

Many authors highlight the "relative subpleural sparing" of the dorsal lower lobe regions as an interesting CT feature to distinguish fibrotic NSIP from UIP (seen in about 20-65% of patients) [1, 15].

Lymph node enlargement has been reported in almost 80% of cases.

CT characteristics of NSIP change over time.

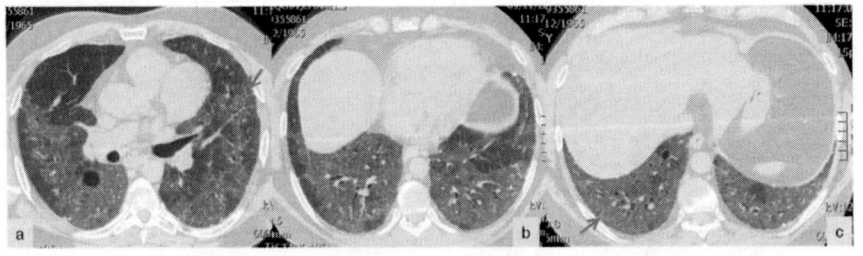

Figure 6. Cellular NSIP: Axial high-resolution CT images: scattered ground glass opacities with a basal and symmetric distribution (red arrow) accompanied by bronchiectasis (blue arrow). Honeycombing is absent.

In fact, CT findings in cellular NSIP may improve or be resolved after treatment in contrast with fibrotic NSIP which is a severe evolutive disease closely resembling UIP.

Acute exacerbation is less common in NSIP than in UIP [8, 16].

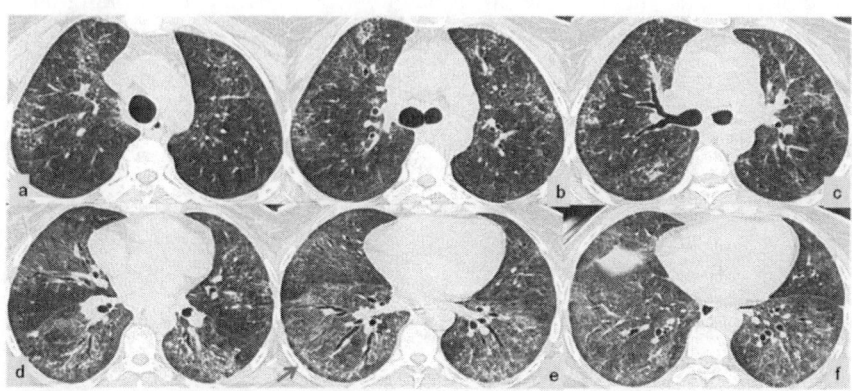

Figure 7. Axial high resolution CT images (NSIP pattern): ground glass opacities associated with irregular septal thickening, bronchovascular distortion. These features have a symmetric distribution and basal medullar predominance. Note the subpleural sparing (blue arrow).

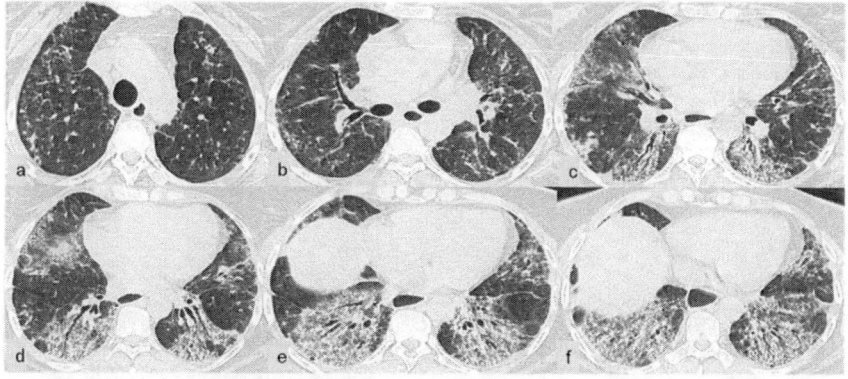

Figure 8. Same patient follow-up CT 2 years later. Axial HRCT images show a clear increase of fibrosis signs: reticulations, bronchiectasis with an obvious basal distribution and lower lobe volume loss. This ILP was associated with an anti-synthetase syndrome.

The prognosis of NSIP depends on the degree of fibrosis.

Cellular NSIP has a much better prognosis than fibrotic NSIP which has 5-year survival rates ranging from 45% to 90% and 10-year survival rates of only 35% [1].

However, the survival rate for fibrotic NSIP remains better than that of UIP. Most patients with NSIP, particularly cellular NSIP, improve or stabilize with corticosteroid therapy and cytotoxic drugs [16, 18].

3.3. NSIP Associated with CTD

NSIP is the most common histopathologic and high-resolution CT pattern of ILD seen in patients with CTD. It is particularly prevalent in progressive systemic sclerosis, polymyositis/dermatomyositis (PM/DM), and mixed connective tissue disease.

It may precede the diagnosis of collagen vascular disease by months or years. For this reason, evidence of underlying collagen vascular disease should be sought both at the initial diagnosis of biopsy-proven NSIP and during the follow-up period, even in the absence of systemic symptoms, especially in young patients [18].

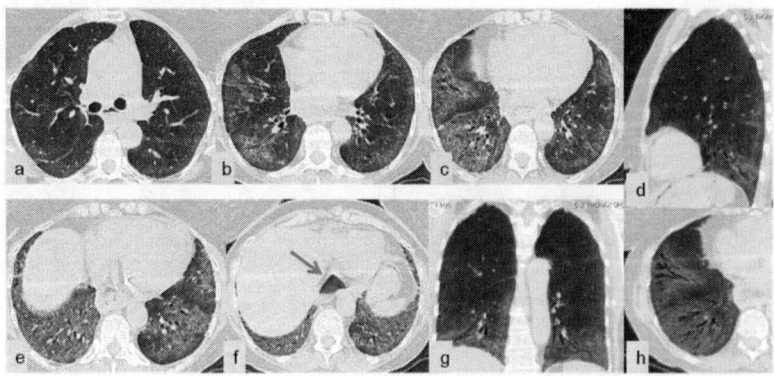

Figure 9. (a, b, c, e, f): axial HR-CT, d, g and h: sagittal, coronal and axial minimal intensity projection reconstructions. Bilateral symmetric areas of ground glass opacities with significant bronchial distortion. These features predominate in the lower lobes sparing the dorsal subpleural layer. Note the dilated esophagus (blue arrow): NSIP associated with scleroderma.

High-resolution CT findings are identical to those seen in idiopathic NSIP. However, every extra-pulmonary semiologic sign should be carefully examined; a dilated thoracic esophagus for example may suggest a diagnosis of scleroderma [18].

The mortality rate is similar among patients with NSIP idiopathic or associated connective tissue disease [18, 19].

4. ORGANIZING PNEUMONIA

Organizing pneumonia is a nonspecific inflammatory response by the lung to different agents such as infection, inhalation injury, drugs, or radiation therapy.

It may also occur in association with inflammatory bowel disease or collagen vascular disease.

In some cases, no underlying cause is identified; the interstitial lung pneumonia is qualified as "cryptogenic organizing pneumonia" [1].

Upon histologic examination, organizing pneumonia is patchy, characterized by an airspace-filling fibroblastic proliferation. It involves alveolar ducts with or without bronchiolar intraluminal polyps.

This pattern is associated with various degrees of edema and inflammatory cell infiltration.

Typically, the lung architecture is preserved [20–22].

4.1. CT Features

4.1.1. Classic Form

4.1.1.1. Multifocal Parenchymal Consolidation
A radiologic examination (chest X-ray and CT scanner) commonly reveals subpleural and/or peribronchovascular consolidation areas with air bronchogram signs.

They may organize as thick radial bands (>8 mm) extending towards the pleura or as curvilinear bands parallel to the pleura.

Areas of traction bronchiectasis may be found as well as ground glass opacities.

These features are often bilateral with asymmetric distribution.

Lung consolidations are often migratory; they may disappear spontaneously while new areas of consolidation appear in different places.

Some studies reported predominance in the lower lobes [23].

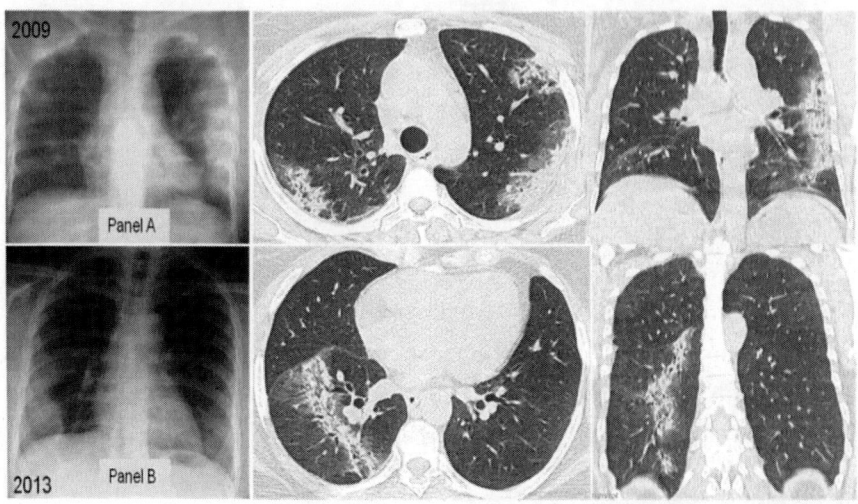

Figure 10. Panel A: chest X-Ray: left peripheric alveolar opacity; HRCT: bilateral subpleural consolidations, Panel B: chest X-Ray: right sided alveolar opacity: HRCT: disappearance of left pulmonary condensations and emergence of pleura to pleura lower lobe consolidation.

4.1.2. Unusual Patterns

4.1.2.1. Reversed Halo Sign

A reversed halo or atoll sign is defined by the presence of a focal area of ground glass opacities or normal lung surrounded by a crescent or ring of consolidation. Initially, it was considered pathognomonic for COP, but it is now admitted that this sign is not specific seen in other diseases including infection, lymphomatoid granulomatosis, or granulomatosis with polyangiitis.

Nevertheless, this sign may also reflect a histological lung reaction of OP associated with or secondary to these various etiologies [24].

4.1.2.2. Perilobular Abnormalities

This imaging finding consists of bowed or polygonal opacities with poorly defined margins surrounding the interlobular septa. They are observed in about half of patients and are often accompanied by consolidation and/or GGO in the same lung zone [24].

This pattern may be explained by the fact that, in the healing phase of the disease, the pulmonary lobule is cleared centripetally involving perilobular areas and mimicking septal abnormalities on CT.

Real septal thickening may also be associated [22].

4.1.2.3. Nodules and Masses

A high-resolution CT scan may reveal solid, mixed density or ground glass nodules in 15 to 50% of OP [17, 22].

These nodules do not have a specific distribution and are either scattered or peribroncho vascular. They may have spiculated borders making it difficult to distinguish from a neoplasm.

Excavation was rarely reported [17].

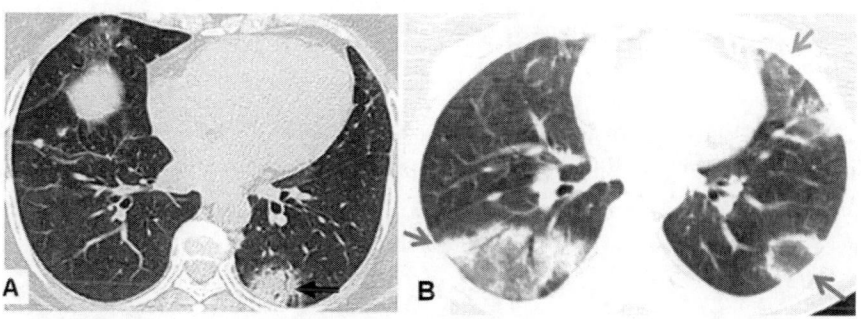

Figure 11. Unusual patterns of OP: HRCT axial images: A: nodular and pseudotumoral consolidation (black arrow) B: reversed Halo sign (blue arrow), peri bronchial consolidation (red arrow) and ground glass opacities (green arrow).

4.2. OP Associated with CTD

The most common CVD associated with OP is PM/DM.

However, OP is the second most common form of ILD in PM/DM after NSIP.

OP also occurs with increased frequency in rheumatoid arthritis (RA) and has been described in systemic lupus erythematosus (SLE) and in Sjögren syndrome [25].

Patients usually respond well to corticosteroid therapy and have a good prognosis. However, patients with OP associated with CTD seem to have a greater risk of relapse and develop fibrosis more often than patients with cryptogenic OP [26].

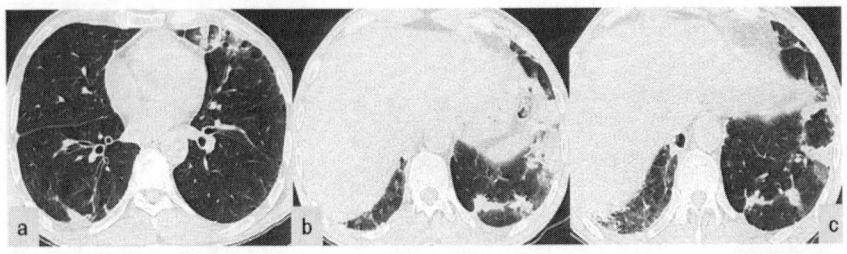

Figure 12. OP in patient treated for RA. Subpleural and peri bronchiolar condensations associated with ground glass opacities in both lungs.

5. Smoking-Related Interstitial Lung Disease

According to the American Thoracic Society/European Respiratory Society statement published in 2013, the term Smoking-Related Interstitial Lung Disease incorporates most cases of DIP, nearly all cases of RB-ILD and Langerhans' cell histiocytosis.

Since this statement was released, many studies have revealed that smokers are at a higher risk of developing chronic fibrosing lung diseases such as Airspace enlargement with fibrosis (AEF), combined pulmonary fibrosis and emphysema (CPFE), usual interstitial pneumonia (UIP), non-specific interstitial pneumonia (NSIP) and other unclassifiable interstitial pneumonia due to the overlap of histological and radiological features in the smoker's lung [3, 27].

5.1. Respiratory Bronchiolitis-Interstitial Lung Disease (RB-ILD)

RB is a common histological lesion seen in smokers. The majority of cases of RB are asymptomatic. It is characterized by pigmented macrophage accumulation within respiratory bronchioles.

RB-ILD is a clinical condition encountered when respiratory bronchiolitis is extensive enough to cause symptoms and show evidence of ILD.

Histological findings of RB-ILD include RB and peribronchiolar fibrosis.

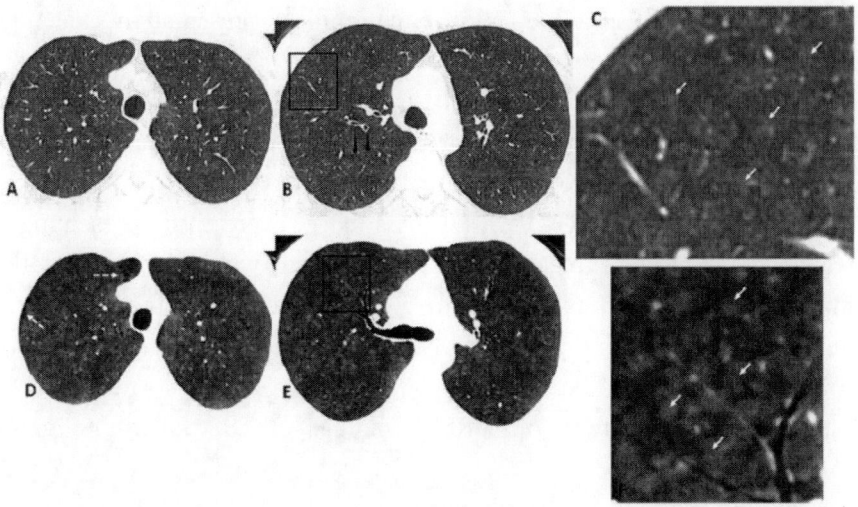

Figure 13. Fortuitous finding of respiratory bronchiolitis in a heavy smoker patient (a, b, c) axial reconstructions, (d, e, f) minimal intensity projection reconstructions centrilobular nodules and ground-glass opacities (arrows), with emphysematous areas (dashed arrows) and bronchial wall thickening (arrowheads).

A chest X-ray is often normal. On HRCT images, centrilobular nodules and ground glass opacities are the predominant abnormalities in RB.

Bronchiolar wall thickening has been also reported in RB-ILD.

Some authors described the upper lobes to be predominately affected.

These patterns usually regress after the patient quits smoking with or without treatment [27–29].

5.2. Desquamative Interstitial Pneumonia

DIP is a rare form of interstitial pneumonia which is usually but not always associated with smoking [29].

The term DIP remains in use due to convention, but is a misnomer, as the alveolar infiltrate represents alveolar macrophage accumulation rather than alveolar desquamation [30].

It is classified separately from RB-ILD according to the latest ATS classification because it has a different clinical presentation, imaging findings, and treatment response [20].

Histological hallmarks of DIP include prominent intra-alveolar accumulation of macrophages, hyperplasia of type II pneumocytes, and, more variably, diffuse alveolar septal thickening.

In comparison with RB-ILD, DIP is a more severe entity presenting a greater extent of lesions (macrophages seen diffusely within the acini in DIP, unlike RB-ILD which is limited to a bronchocentric distribution) and interstitial fibrosis with possible lymphoid follicles and eosinophilic infiltration [27].

The dominant pattern on HRCT findings of DIP is ground glass opacities.

They are reported to have lower zone predominance with subpleural distribution.

Random and diffuse distributions have also been described.

A basal reticular pattern associated with irregular linear opacities is a common marker of fibrosis seen in DIP.

Small cystic airspaces, different from honeycombing lesions, may be present in areas of ground glass opacity [20].

The main radiological difference between RB-associated ILD and DIP is the distribution of disease: centrilobular nodules are uncommon in DIP while ground glass opacities are usually patchier and less extensive in RB-associated ILD [1].

5.3. Pulmonary Langerhans Cell Histiocytosis

Pulmonary Langerhans cell histiocytosis is a form of LCH strongly associated with_smoking. In fact, more than 90% of patients are either current or previous smokers.

Patients are usually young adults (men or women) aged from 20 to 40 years.

Extrapulmonary manifestations are rare, occurring in about 5-10% of patients. High resolution computed tomography (HRCT) demonstrates small, ill-defined centrilobular nodules which are the earliest radiological signs. Nodules are the infiltration of Langerhans cells centered in small airways. The nodules may enlarge and cavitate, forming cysts. As the disease progresses, the cysts coalesce and become irregularly shaped, classically described as "bizarre" shaped.

Findings are predominately seen in the upper lung zones with relative sparing of the bases. HRCT findings are characteristic of the disease so that ung biopsy is usually unnecessary. Smoking cessation can lead to clinical improvement with a clearly better prognosis [29, 31, 32].

Nodules and micronodules (blue arrow) associated with cystic lesions (red arrow) and irregular septal thickening. These features are bilateral involving both cortical and medullar pulmonary regions with upper lobe predominance.

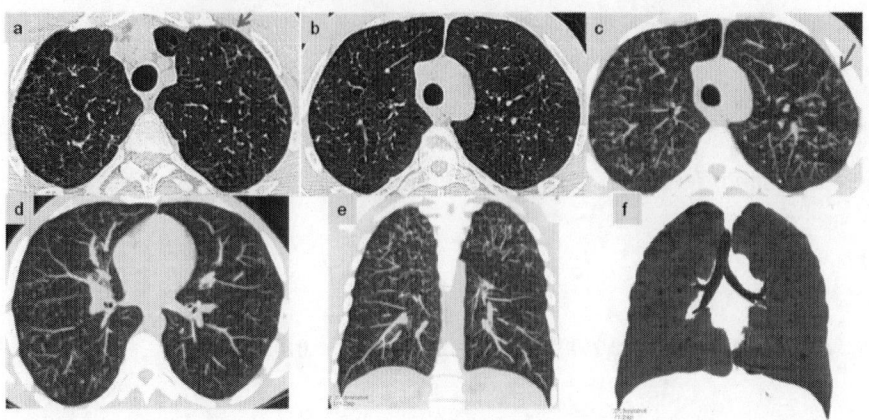

Figure 14. (a,b) HRCT axial images. (c,d,e) maximum intensity projection axial and coronal reconstructions; (f) minimum intensity projection coronal reconstruction.

5.4. Airspace Enlargement with Fibrosis (AEF) and Combined Pulmonary Fibrosis and Emphysema (CPFE)

Emphysema is characterized by permanently enlarged distal airspaces without obvious fibrosis.

However, and especially in heavy smokers, signs of fibrosis are often present in histologic specimens.

Thus, the term air space enlargement with fibrosis was proposed in 2006 and 2008 to represent the histological findings of fibrosis coexisting with emphysema [33, 34].

It presents on an HRCT scanner as thin-walled cysts contrasting with imperceptible walls surrounding lesions in typical emphysema.

A pattern of cystic spaces within reticulations was also described in AEF scanner findings [32, 35].

Combined pulmonary fibrosis and emphysema (CPFE) is a clinical condition reflecting the presence of both fibrosing lesions and emphysema in the same patient.

On HRCT, CPFE is characterized by the coexistence of emphysema in upper zones and patterns of interstitial fibrosing pneumonia in the lower lobes including AEF, NSIP or UIP [32].

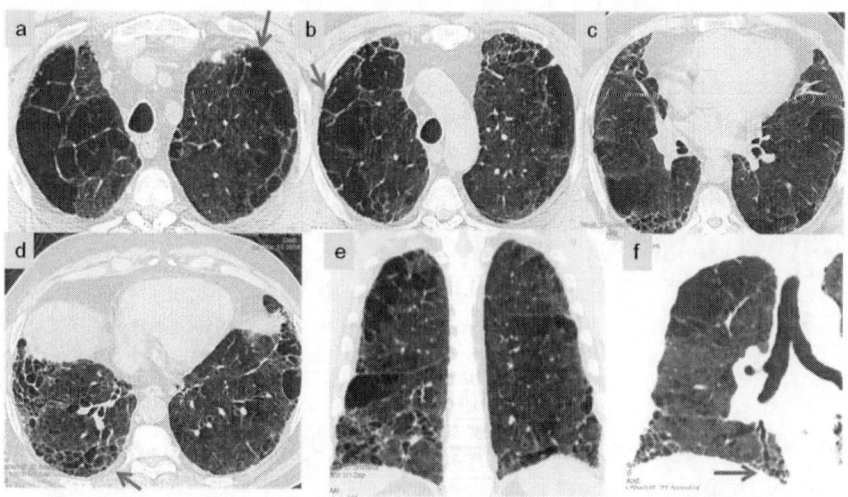

Figure 15. Combined pulmonary fibrosis and emphysema (CPFE): axial (a, b, c, d) and coronal (e, f) reconstructions showing emphysema in the upper lobes (blue arrows) and pulmonary fibrosis in the lower lobes (red arrows) (honeycombing lesions, traction bronchiectasis and reticular opacities).

6. LYMPHOCYTIC INTERSTITIAL PNEUMONIA

Lymphocytic interstitial pneumonia (LIP) is a rare clinicopathologic condition involving an inflammatory pulmonary reaction of the bronchus-associated lymphoid tissue (BALT).

Its pathological mechanism is an interstitial infiltration by reactive T and B lymphocytes, plasma cells, and histiocytes [36].

LIP must be distinguished from low grade malignant lymphoproliferative diseases by immunohistochemical analysis although the risk of malignant transformation is low, estimated at about 5% [1].

Idiopathic LIP is very rare. It is much more commonly associated with CTD, auto immune conditions, acquired immunodeficiency syndrome and other immunodeficiencies.

Among CTDs, LIP is most closely associated with SS but also with SLE and RA [10, 36].

6.1. HRCT Features

The HRCT features consist of patchy or confluent bilateral ground glass opacities associated with centrilobular and subpleural micronodules [36].

Interlobular septal thickening and thickened bronchovascular bundles have also been reported [20].

These features predominate in the lower lobes.

Thin-walled cysts (1–30 mm), usually few in number, are a hallmark feature of LIP disease.

Cyst formation has been explicated by a valve mechanism involving small bronchioles being obstructed or partially obstructed by the adjacent lymphocyte infiltration.

Well- or ill-defined larger nodules may occasionally be seen in patients with LIP; these are usually amyloid deposits which may calcify. An associated lymphoma must be first ruled out. Enlarged adenopathy may also be seen [25].

7. PLEUROPARENCHYMAL FIBROELASTOSIS

PPFE is a rare condition classified as a rare IIP. It consists of a fibrosing process rich in elastic fibers involving the pleura and subpleural lung parenchyma. It predominates in the upper lobes [3].

Although the etiology of PPFE is considered idiopathic in most cases, it has been reported to be associated with some factors such as genetic predisposition, recurrent lower respiratory tract infections, collagen vascular diseases, bone marrow transplantation or lung transplantation restrictive allograft syndrome [37].

HRCT shows irregular pleural thickening, dense subpleural consolidation with traction bronchiectasis, architectural distortion, and upper lobe volume loss.

Differential diagnoses include fibrotic sarcoidosis, hypersensitivity pneumonitis, and connective tissue disease, particularly ankylosing spondylitis.

Thus, the final diagnosis is made through a lung biopsy [20].

Conclusion

The interstitial pneumonias are a heterogeneous group of diffuse parenchymal lung diseases with diverse imaging manifestations, clinical features, and outcomes. They may be idiopathic or secondary to other disorders such as connective tissue diseases.

Imaging techniques, especially high-resolution computed tomography, are the main diagnostic tools.

HRCT makes positive diagnosis of interstitial pneumonias possible and, in most cases, classifies them according to the latest international Multidisciplinary Classification.

It also aims to find associated signs which may lead to suspicions of an associated connective tissue disease.

Using this imaging technique, a patient's prognosis can be evaluated and followed up.

Although HR-CT is a cornerstone in diagnosing interstitial pneumonias, a multidisciplinary approach is mandatory for the best patient management.

References

[1] Ferguson, E. C., Berkowitz, E. A. (2012). Lung CT: Part 2, The Interstitial Pneumonias: Clinical, Histologic, and CT Manifestations. *Am J Roentgenol,* Oct;199(4):W464–76.

[2] American Thoracic Society/European Respiratory Society International Multidisciplinary Consensus Classification of the Idiopathic Interstitial Pneumonias: This Joint Statement of the

American Thoracic Society (ATS), and the European Respiratory Society (ERS) was adopted by the ATS Board of Directors, June 2001 and by The ERS Executive Committee, June 2001. *Am J Respir Crit Care Med.* 2002 Jan 15;165(2):277–304.

[3] Travis, W. D., Costabel, U., Hansell, D. M., King, T. E., Lynch, D. A., Nicholson, A. G., et al. (2013). An Official American Thoracic Society/European Respiratory Society Statement: Update of the International Multidisciplinary Classification of the Idiopathic Interstitial Pneumonias. *Am J Respir Crit Care Med*, Sep 15;188 (6):733–48.

[4] Raghu G, Remy-Jardin M, Myers JL, Richeldi L, Ryerson CJ, Lederer DJ, et al. (2018). Diagnosis of Idiopathic Pulmonary Fibrosis. An Official ATS/ERS/JRS/ALAT Clinical Practice Guideline. *Am J Respir Crit Care Med,* Sep;198(5):e44–68.

[5] Kusmirek, J. E., Martin, M. D., Kanne, J. P. (2016). Imaging of Idiopathic Pulmonary Fibrosis. *Radiol Clin North Am*, Nov;54(6):997–1014.

[6] Salvatore, M., Smith, M. L. (2018). Cross sectional imaging of pulmonary fibrosis translating pathology into radiology. *Clin Imaging*, Sep; 51:332–6.

[7] Lynch, D. A., Sverzellati, N., Travis, W. D., Brown, K. K., Colby, T. V., Galvin, J. R., et al. (2018). Diagnostic criteria for idiopathic pulmonary fibrosis: a Fleischner Society White Paper. *Lancet Respir Med*, Feb;6(2):138–53.

[8] Silva, C. I. S., Müller, N. L., Fujimoto, K., Kato, S., Ichikado, K., Taniguchi, H., et al. (2007). Acute exacerbation of chronic interstitial pneumonia: high-resolution computed tomography and pathologic findings. *J Thorac Imaging*, Aug;22(3):221–9.

[9] Kim, E. A., Lee, K. S., Johkoh, T., Kim, T. S., Suh, G. Y., Kwon, O. J., et al. (2002). Interstitial lung diseases associated with collagen vascular diseases: radiologic and histopathologic findings. *Radiogr Rev Publ Radiol Soc N Am Inc*, Oct;22 Spec No:S151-165.

[10] Henry, T. S., Little, B. P., Veeraraghavan, S., Bhalla, S., Elicker, B. M. (2016). The Spectrum of Interstitial Lung Disease in Connective Tissue Disease. *J Thorac Imaging*, Mar;31(2):65–77.

[11] Bryson, T., Sundaram, B., Khanna, D., Kazerooni, E. A. (2014). Connective Tissue Disease–Associated Interstitial Pneumonia and Idiopathic Interstitial Pneumonia: Similarity and Difference. *Semin Ultrasound CT MRI*, Feb;35(1):29–38.

[12] Ruano, C. A., Lucas, R. N., Leal, C. I., Lourenço, J., Pinheiro, S., Fernandes, O., et al. (2015). Thoracic Manifestations of Connective Tissue Diseases. *Curr Probl Diagn Radiol*, Jan;44(1):47–59.

[13] Chung, J. H., Cox, C. W., Montner, S. M., Adegunsoye, A., Oldham, J. M., Husain, A. N., et al. (2018). CT Features of the Usual Interstitial Pneumonia Pattern: Differentiating Connective Tissue Disease–Associated Interstitial Lung Disease From Idiopathic Pulmonary Fibrosis. *Am J Roentgenol*, Feb;210(2):307–13.

[14] Gruden, J. F. (2016). CT in Idiopathic Pulmonary Fibrosis: Diagnosis and Beyond. *Am J Roentgenol*, Mar;206(3):495–507.

[15] Travis, W. D., Hunninghake, G., King, T. E., Lynch, D. A., Colby, T. V., Galvin, J. R,. et al. (2008). Idiopathic Nonspecific Interstitial Pneumonia: Report of an American Thoracic Society Project. *Am J Respir Crit Care Med*, Jun 15;177(12):1338–47.

[16] Kligerman, S. J., Groshong, S., Brown, K. K., Lynch, D. A. (2009). Nonspecific Interstitial Pneumonia: Radiologic, Clinical, and Pathologic Considerations. *RadioGraphics*, Jan;29(1):73–87.

[17] Neji, H., Attia, M., Affes, M., Baccouche, I., Ben Miled-M'rad, K., Hantous-Zannad, S. (2018). Interstitial lung diseases: Imaging contribution to diagnosis and elementary radiological lesions. *Semin Diagn Pathol*, Sep;35(5):297–303.

[18] Capobianco, J., Grimberg, A., Thompson, B. M., Antunes, V. B., Jasinowodolinski D., Meirelles G. S. P. (2012). Thoracic Manifestations of Collagen Vascular Diseases. *RadioGraphics*, Jan;32(1):33–50.

[19] Tansey, D., Wells, A. U., Colby, T. V., Ip, S., Nikolakoupolou, A., du Bois, R. M., et al. (2004). Variations in histological patterns of

interstitial pneumonia between connective tissue disorders and their relationship to prognosis. *Histopathology*, Jun;44(6):585–96.

[20] Sverzellati, N., Lynch, D. A., Hansell, D. M., Johkoh, T., King, T. E., Travis, W. D. (2015). American Thoracic Society–European Respiratory Society Classification of the Idiopathic Interstitial Pneumonias: Advances in Knowledge since 2002. *RadioGraphics*, Nov;35(7): 1849–71.

[21] Oliveira, D. S., Araújo Filho, J de A., Paiva, A. F. L., Ikari, E. S., Chate, R. C., Nomura, C. H.(2018). Idiopathic interstitial pneumonias: review of the latest American Thoracic Society/European Respiratory Society classification. *Radiol Bras*, Oct 18;51(5):321–7.

[22] Zare, Mehrjardi M., Kahkouee, S., Pourabdollah, M. (2017). Radio-Pathological Correlation of Organising Pneumonia (OP): A Pictorial Review. *Br J Radiol*, Jan 20;20160723.

[23] Baque-Juston, M., Pellegrin, A., Leroy, S., Marquette, C. H., Padovani, B. (2014). Organizing pneumonia: What is it? A conceptual approach and pictorial review. *Diagn Interv Imaging*, Sep;95(9):771–7.

[24] Torrealba, J. R., Fisher, S., Kanne, J. P., Butt, Y. M., Glazer, C., Kershaw, C., et al. (2018). Pathology-radiology correlation of common and uncommon computed tomographic patterns of organizing pneumonia. *Hum Pathol*, Jan; 71:30–40.

[25] Silva CIS, Müller NL. (2010). Interstitial Lung Disease in the Setting of Collagen Vascular Disease. *Semin Roentgenol*, Jan;45(1):22–8.

[26] Chung, M. P., Nam, B. D., Lee, K. S., Han, J., Park, J. S., Hwang, J. H., et al. (2018). Serial chest CT in cryptogenic organizing pneumonia: Evolutional changes and prognostic determinants: Serial CT and prognostic factor in COP. *Respirology*, Mar;23(3):325–30.

[27] Iwasawa, T., Takemura, T., Ogura, T. (2018). Smoking-related lung abnormalities on computed tomography images: comparison with pathological findings. *Jpn J Radiol*, Mar;36(3):165–80.

[28] Sieminska, A., Kuziemski, K. (2014). Respiratory bronchiolitis-interstitial lung disease. *Orphanet J Rare Dis*, Dec; 9(1). Available

from: http://ojrd.biomedcentral.com/articles/10.1186/s13023-014010 6-8.

[29] Cheng, S, Mohammed, T. L. H. (2015). Diffuse Smoking-Related Lung Disease: Emphysema and Interstitial Lung Disease. *Semin Roentgenol*, Jan;50(1):16–22.

[30] Fromm, G. B., Dunn, L. J., Ocie Harris, J.(1980). Desquamative Interstitial Pneumonitis. *Chest*, Apr;77(4):552–4.

[31] Nair, A., Hansell, D. M. (2014). High-Resolution Computed Tomography Features of Smoking-Related Interstitial Lung Disease. *Semin Ultrasound CT MRI*, Feb;35(1):59–71.

[32] Madan, R., Matalon, S., Vivero, M. (2016). Spectrum of Smoking-related Lung Diseases: Imaging Review and Update. *J Thorac Imaging*, Mar;31(2):78–91.

[33] Yousem, S. A. (2006) Respiratory bronchiolitis-associated interstitial lung disease with fibrosis is a lesion distinct from fibrotic nonspecific interstitial pneumonia: a proposal. *Mod Pathol*, Nov;19(11):1474–9.

[34] Kawabata, Y., Hoshi, E., Murai, K., Ikeya, T., Takahashi, N., Saitou, Y., et al. (2008). Smoking-related changes in the background lung of specimens resected for lung cancer: a semiquantitative study with correlation to postoperative course. *Histopathology*, Dec;53(6):707–14.

[35] Margaritopoulos, G. A., Vasarmidi, E., Jacob, J., Wells, A. U., Antoniou, K. M. (2015). Smoking and interstitial lung diseases. *Eur Respir Rev*, Sep;24(137):428–35.

[36] Sirajuddin, A., Raparia, K., Lewis, V. A., Franks, T. J., Dhand, S., Galvin, J. R., et al. (2016). Primary Pulmonary Lymphoid Lesions: Radiologic and Pathologic Findings. *RadioGraphics*, Jan;36(1):53–70.

[37] Esteves, C., Costa, F. R., Redondo, M. T., Moura, C. S., Guimarães, S., Morais, A., et al. (2016) . Pleuroparenchymal fibroelastosis: role of high-resolution computed tomography (HRCT) and CT-guided transthoracic core lung biopsy. *Insights Imaging*, Feb;7(1):155–62.

In: Interstitial Lung Disease
Editor: Liva T. Villadsen

ISBN: 978-1-53616-246-2
© 2019 Nova Science Publishers, Inc.

Chapter 4

LUNG SARCOIDOSIS: TYPICAL AND ATYPICAL FEATURES ON COMPUTED TOMOGRAPHY

Henda Nèji[1,3],*MD, Monia Attia[1,3]MD,
Mariem Affes[1,3]MD,
Houda Gharsalli[2,3] MD, Ines Baccouche[1]MD,
Khaoula Ben Miled-M'rad[1,3]MD,
and Saoussen Hantous-Zannad[1,3] MD

[1]Imaging Department
[2]"D" Pulmonology Department
Abderrahmen Mami Hospital, Ariana, Tunisia,
[3]Faculty of Medicine of Tunis, Tunis El Manar University,
Tunis, Tunisia

---

* Corresponding Author's Email: hendaneji@gmail.com.

Abstract

Sarcoidosis is a systemic granulomatous disease which involves the lungs in more than 90% of cases. It is one of the leading causes of interstitial involvement in lung diseases. Its diagnosis is based on compatible clinical, biological, imaging and anatomopathological features. Thus, imaging is considered to be a cornerstone in the work-up and follow-up of the disease. High-resolution computed tomography (HR-CT) is more sensitive and more accurate than plain chest radiography in diagnosing parenchymal involvement.

In the inflammatory active forms, CT, typically shows micronodules of perilymphatic distribution, involving, the bronchovascular bundle, interlobular septa and fissures. In the fibrotic forms, patients present with one of three different patterns: bronchial distortion with or without central pseudo-masses, honeycombing or an irregular linear pattern. Classically, all these features are bilateral, symmetric, and involve the upper, mid and posterior parts of the lungs.

Atypical presentations include nodules and masses with irregular margins, alveolar consolidations, excavations, ground glass opacities, predominant septal thickening, miliary appearance, large and small airways involvement with air trapping. Features may be also distributed in an atypical manner to one side or to the lower parts of the lungs.

Radiological diagnosis is often easy in typical forms but may be challenging in some cases. Excluding lung cancer, carcinomatous lymphangitis and necrotizing as well as mycobacterial infections may sometimes be necessary.

Keywords: sarcoidosis, lung, computed tomography, inflammation, fibrosis

1. Introduction

Sarcoïdosis is a systemic inflammatory disease of unknown etiology despite the attempts to link it to exposure to mycobacterial antigens [1, 2]. Histologically, this disease is characterized by the presence of granuloma without caseous necrosis, thus differentiating it from tuberculosis. The most involved areas are the lungs and mediastinum. Patients may be symptomatic or asymptomatic. Sarcoidosis is diagnosed by gathering clinical, biological, radiological and histological arguments. A chest X-ray, which can be normal or abnormal, is the first radiographic exam to be done. High resolution computed tomography (HR-CT) is considered to be the most sensitive imaging tool in diagnosing parenchymal involvement. CT features of lung sarcoidosis vary widely. They can be typical, making the diagnosis easy, or atypical suggesting other diseases.

2. CHEST HR-CT INDICATIONS IN SARCOIDOSIS

A multidetector CT makes it possible to explore the whole chest exploration in a single breath-hold with 0.5 to 1.2mm slice thickness. However, an interspaced HR-CT may be preferable in young patients to reduce exposure to irradiation [3].

HR-CT indications are controversial. In fact, despite its superiority to chest X-ray, only 30% of patient have this exploration done in the work up of their disease [4]. Some indications, however, still recommend the use of HR-CT according to the American Thoracic society (ATS)/European Respiratory Society (ERS)/World Association of Sarcoidosis and Other Granulomatous Disorders (WASOG) expert consensus statement on sarcoidosis. These include atypical clinical and/or radiographic features, discord between clinical and radiographic findings and a complications assessment [4, 5, 6]. CT may also be indicated before transbronchial biopsy, bronchoalveolar lavage or surgical biopsy. Moreover, CT is valuable for prognosis because it distinguishes between reversible (active inflammation) and irreversible (fibrosis) disease. Therefore, it can predict the response to anti-inflammatory treatment [7]. Despite all these advantages, the extent of CT features does not correlate with functional and bronchoalveolar lavage tests results [4]. How the disease will be be followed up and for how long are not consensual either [5].

3. Typical Lung CT Features in Sarcoïdosis

3.1. Active Inflammatory Form

Typically, in its active forms, perilymphatic micronodules along the bronchovascular bundle, interlobular septa, interlobar fissures and subpleural regions are the hallmark of the disease [4, 8]. They are found in 80 to 100% of patients on CT [9]. These micronodules are dense and have well-defined margins. When they are beyond CT resolution, they may appear as ground glass opacities [4, 6]. They result from granulomas agglomerates and they are predominant in the upper-mid and posterior lungs (Figure 1). The "galaxy sign" refers to a large nodule with irregular margins that is surrounded by multiple micronodules [5, 10] (Figure 2). "Sarcoïd cluster" corresponds to multiple tiny nodules grouped together [5].

Bronchovascular bundle thickening is another cardinal feature. It usually begins in the hilar regions and may cause bronchial stenosis [5] (Figure 3). In this case, sarcoïdosis should be distinguished from carcinomatous lymphangitis and lymphoma.

3.2. Fibrotic Form

In 10 to 20% of cases, patients evolve toward fibrosis [7]. Fibrotic sarcoïdosis is associated with a high mortality rate that can reach 7.6% [5].

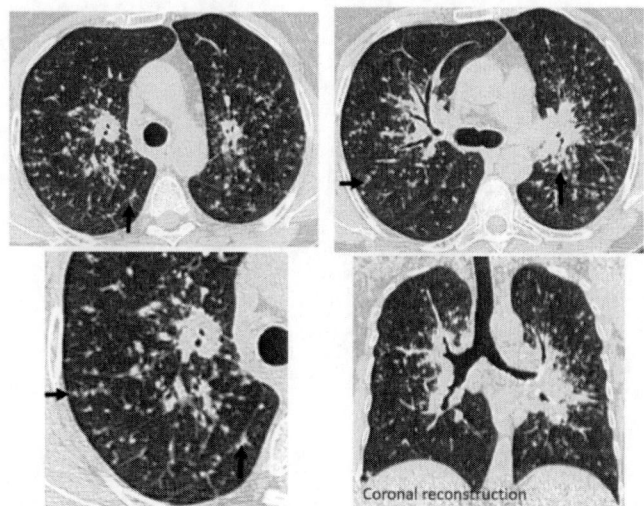

Figure 1. Sarcoïdosis with périlymphatic micronodules along pleura, interlobular septa and bronchovascular bundle, predominating to the mid-upper lungs (arrows).

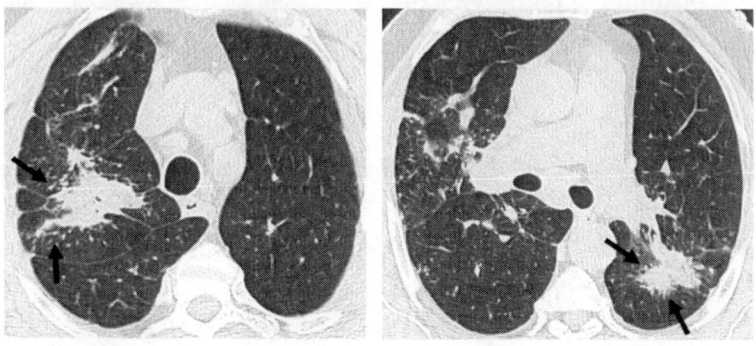

Figure 2. "Galaxy sign": multiple micronodules surrounding masses (arrows).

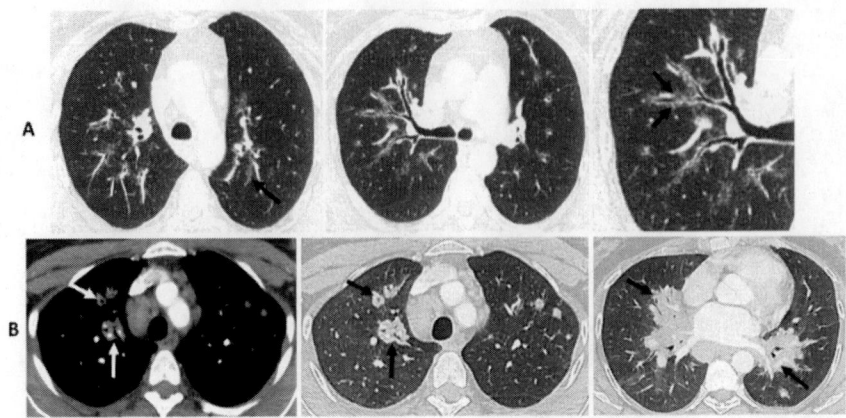

Figure 3. (Panel A): Peribronchovascular bundle thickening with "ground glass" appearance (arrows). (Panel B): Proximal and distal tissular peribronchovascular bundle thickening (arrows).

In the fibrotic forms, patients present with one of three different patterns: bronchial distortion with or without central pseudo-masses, honeycombing or an irregular linear pattern [11].

3.2.1. Bronchial Distortion

Bronchial distortion is the most frequent sign. It results from retraction that makes bronchi and vessel displace. Their path is therefore angulated and irregular and their lumen is dilated. The posterior displacement of the right upper lobe bronchus is the most frequent sign of retraction. Bronchiectasis radiate dorsally and laterally from the hilum [6]. The masses of fibrosis predominate in the upper and middle territories and in central perihilar areas [10] (Figure 4). An obstructive pattern is also frequently associated with this condition [12].

3.2.2. Honeycombing

Unlike idiopathic pulmonary fibrosis, honeycombing predominates in the upper and mid lungs [6, 10]. It is described as a cluster of small cystic airspaces and is associated with a restrictive pattern on functional exploration [12] (Figure 5).

3.2.3. Linear Pattern

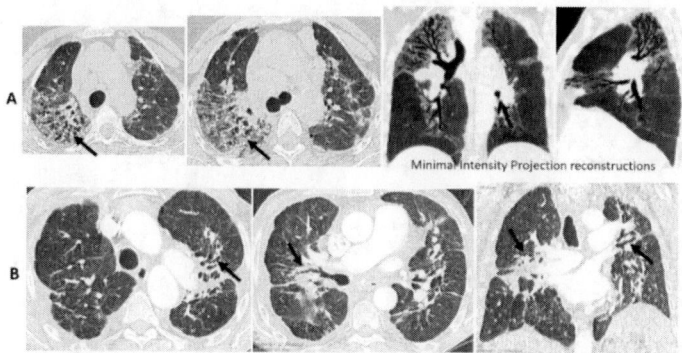

Figure 4. (Panel A): Fibrotic sarcoïdosis with bronchial distortion that is well identified on Minimal Intensity Projection Reconstructions (arrows). (Panel B): Associated fibrotic pseudomasses (arrows).

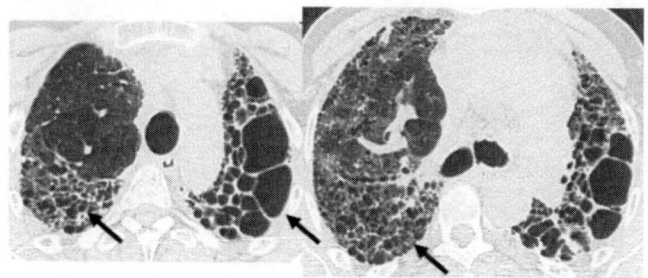

Figure 5. Sarcoïdosis with honeycombing and bullae (arrows).

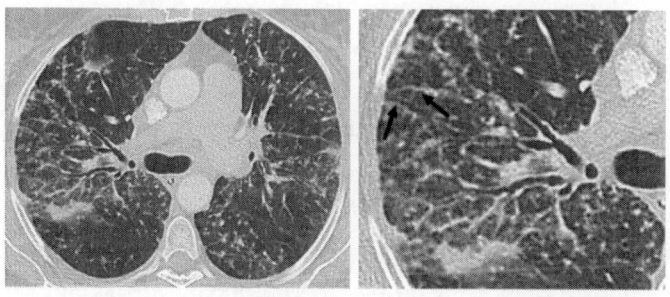

Figure 6. Fibrotic sarcoïdosis with irregular sepetal thickening (arrows).

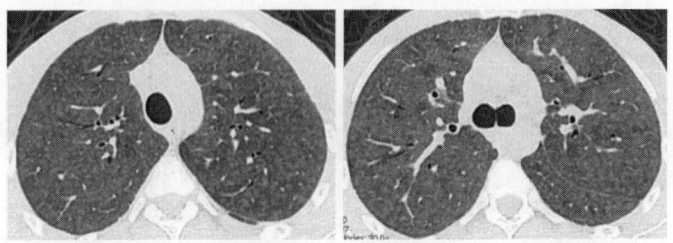

Figure 7. Sarcoïdosis with "ground glass" centrilobular micronodules mimicking hypersensitivity pneumonitis (diagnosis confirmed by surgical biopsy).

Linear pattern includes irregular septal thickening and non-septal lines often with hilar-peripheral lines [10]. Unlike bronchial distortion and honeycombing, this pattern is the most frequently diffused and causes less impairment of the lung function [12] (Figure 6).

4. ATYPICAL LUNG CT FEATURES IN SARCOIDOSIS

There are many atypical features of sarcoïdosis that can lead to misdiagnosis.

4.1. Atypical Distribution of Micronodules

Very rarely, micronodules may have a centrilobular or hematogeneous distribution mimicking hypersensitive pneumonitis, tuberculosis and carcinomatous miliary [5] (Figures 7 and 8). Less than 1% of patients present with a miliary pattern. However, in one recent study, sarcoidosis accounted for 23% of patients with this pattern, which was explained by the frequency of African American patients in the studied population [13]. Attentive examination of CT images shows that the appearance of a miliary pattern more often corresponds to a profuse perilymphatic distribution than to a random one [9]. Coexistence with bilateral enlarged lymph nodes helps with diagnosis [14]. Patients may also present with asymmetrical or unilateral micronodules as well as predominance in lower lungs [8].

4.2. Macronodules and Consolidations

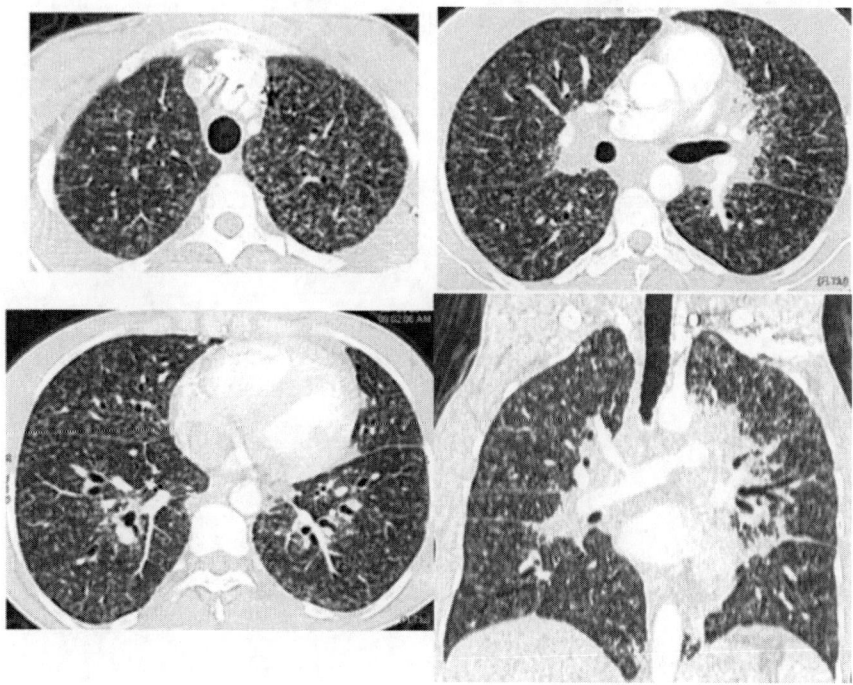

Figure 8. Sarcoïdosis with miliary pattern and random distribution of micronodules (Biopsy: tuberculoïd granulomas with little necrosis. The patient underwent six-month anti-tuberculous treatment with no improvement. Lesions regression was observed after corticotherapy).

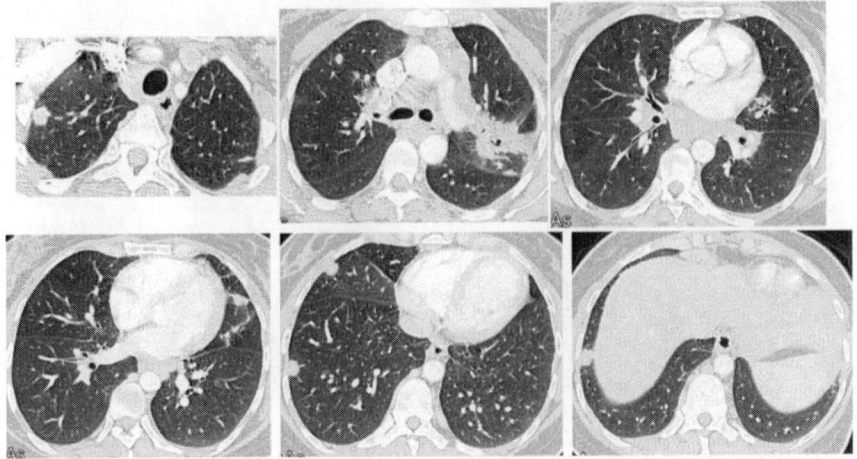

Figure 9. Atypical sarcoïdosis with a culminal mass and bilateral macronodules.

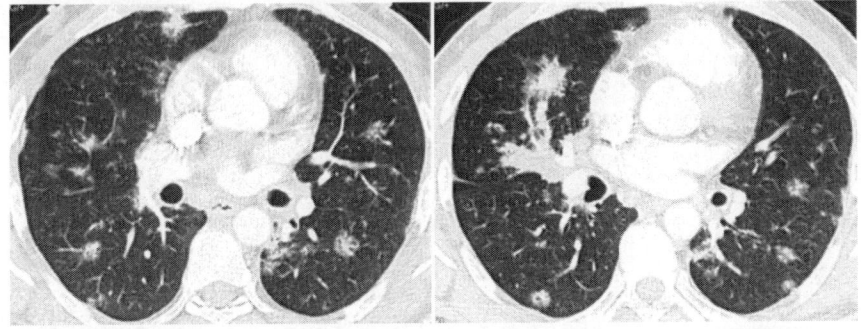

Figure 10. Macronodules with irregular margins.

Macronodules and masses result from coalescence of micronodules. They generally predominate in the mid-upper lung, along the bronchovascular bundle and subpleural areas [5]. The predominance of macronodules/masses and multifocal consolidations is uncommon (Figure 9). Macronodules, masses and consolidations may excavate in 3.4 - 6.8% of cases [10]. Macronodules often present with irregular margins [11] (Figure 10). A reverse halo sign with central ground glass opacity and peripheral consolidation may occasionally be seen [9].

4.3. Cavitary Lesions

Primary excavation in sarcoidosis is uncommon. It occurs in less than 1 - 3% of cases and correlates with an active disease [3, 15, 16]. Patients with cavitary sarcoïdosis are often young with no gender predilection [17]. Necrotizing sarcoidosis is histologically characterized by the presence of vascultitis and non caseating necrosis. Cavities may be present either at the moment of diagnosis or during the follow up with or without treatment [17] (Figure 11). They can be a single cavity or multiple [15]. Co-infection with necrotizing germs such as aspergillosis and tuberculosis should be eliminated before retaining the diagnosis. Cavities should also be distinguished from bullae and cystic bronchiectasis [17]. Erosion of pulmonary arteries by cavitary lesions can be possible and result in hemoptysis [12].

4.4. Bullae

Small and moderate bullae may appear in fibrotic forms. Large bullae invoke "vanishing lung syndrome" (Figure 5). Several theories have been advanced to explain bullae formation including peripheral air trapping and alveolar distension caused by endobronchial disease, destruction of lung tissue by active alveolitis, as well as retraction and collapse of the surrounding lung with air filling of more compliant air spaces [12].

4.5. Ground Glass Opacities

Ground glass opacities are defined as hyperdensities that do not obscure vessels' margins or bronchial walls. They may result from alveolitis or from very small granulomas that are below CT resolution in active disease [12]. They may not disappear when they are in relationship with fibrosis [9] (Figure 12).

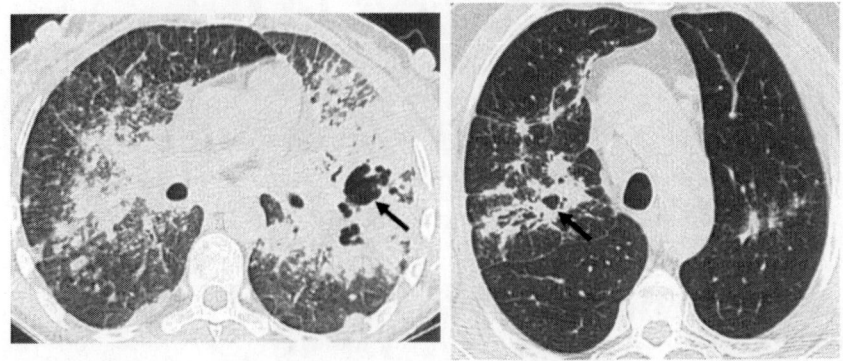

Figure 11. Primary excavation in 2 patients with sarcoïd consolidations (arrows).

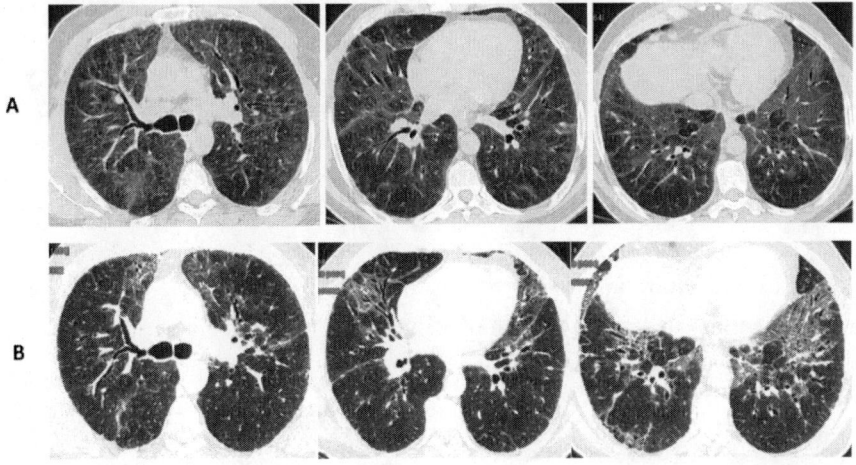

Figure 12. (Panel A): bilateral "ground glass" opacities in a patient with sarcoidosis. (Panel B): Follw up computed tomography showing persistence of these lesions and fibrotic bronchial distorsion.

4.6. Pseudo-Tumoral Presentation

Dominant or solitary mass-like lesions as well as lobar atelectasis due to endobronchial granulomas are uncommon findings. Diagnosis is generally made by transparietal biopsy or after surgical resection [18] (Figures 9 and 13).

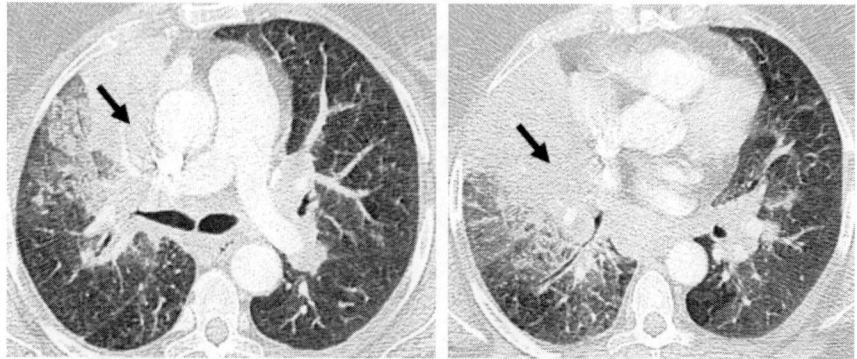

Figure 13. Upper right and middle lobes atelectasis following bronchial obstruction in a pseudo-tumoral sarcoidosis (arrows).

4.7. Airways Involvement and Air Trapping

Large airways are involved in 1 - 3% of cases. Sarcoïd granulomas can cause bronchial stenosis and may be observed in bronchial lumen (Figure 14). Stenosis may be regular, irregular or tumor-like. Tracheobronchomalacia may also be observed [8]. Clustring micronodules around small airways may cause air-trapping and a mosaic appearance on expiratory CT images. This results in an obstructive pattern on functional tests [9] (Figure 15).

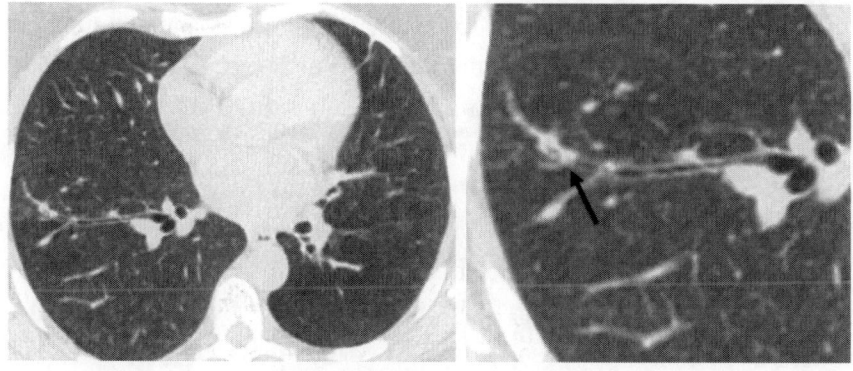

Figure 14. Bronchial involvement with intra-luminal granuloma (arrow).

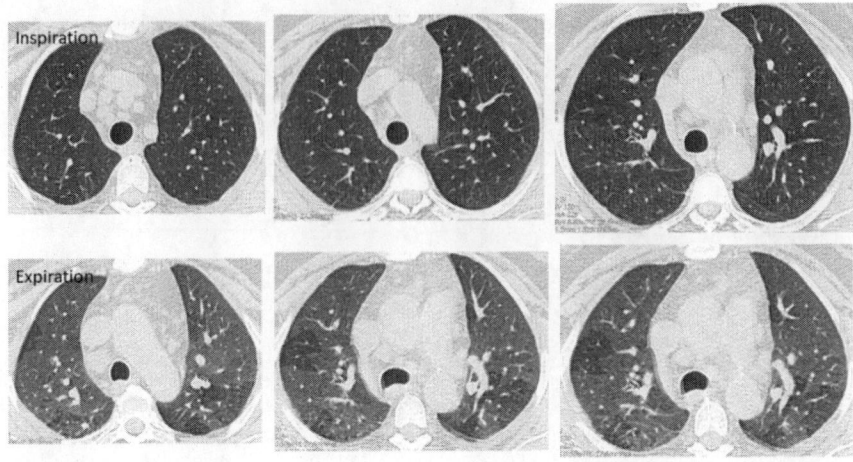

Figure 15. Isolated air trapping in a patient with confirmed sarcoïdosis by mediastinal lymph nodes biopsy.

5. ASSOCIATED SIGNS

5.1. Enlarged Lymph Nodes

CT is more sensitive than chest X-rays in detecting enlarged lymph nodes. They may be seen in 47 - 94% of cases [5]. They are typically large, bilateral (with right predominance), symmetric non-compressive and non-necrotizing, differentiating them from tuberculosis. The most commonly involved stations, in decreasing order are 4R (right lower paratracheal), 10R (right hilar), 7 (sub-carinal), 5 (sub-aortic or aorto-pulmonic window), 11R (right interlobar), and 11 L (left interlobar) [5, 11, 19]. Several stations are usually involved simultaneously. Age, sex and disease stage do not influence their CT pattern [19] (Figure 16). Uncommon presentation include isolated either paratracheal, subcarinal, anterior mediastinal or posterior mediastinal lymphadenopathies [8]. Lymph nodes may be calcified, especially in long-lasting disease (44% at 4 years versus 20% at presentation) [5, 11]. Typically, calcifications are central, amorphous or cloud-like (icing sugar) (Figure 17) but they may also have an egg-shell aspect [5, 20].

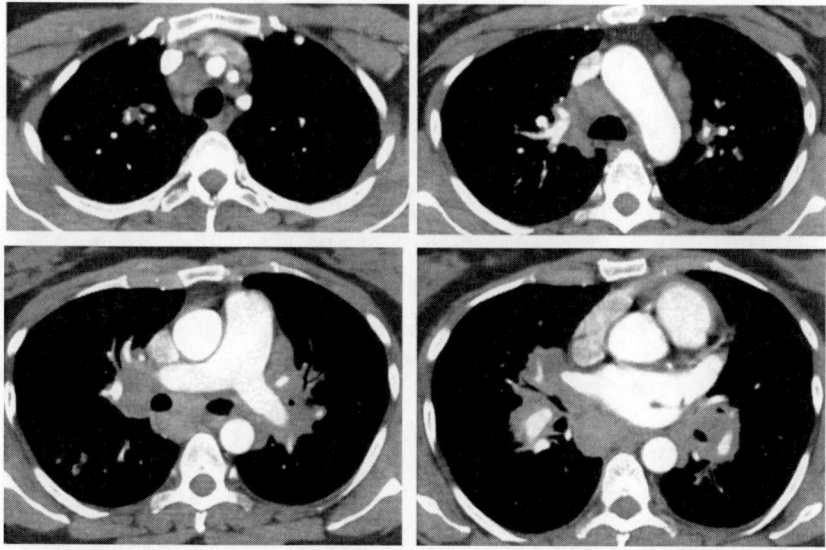

Figure 16. Typical bilateral symmetric and non-compressive mediastinal, hilar and bronchial lymph nodes.

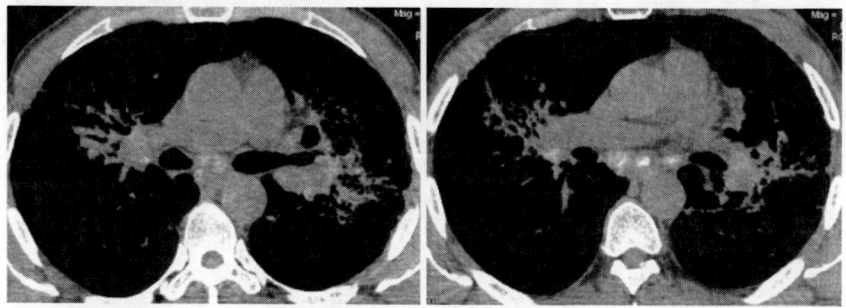

Figure 17. "Icing sugar" calcifications in mediastinal and hilar lymph nodes.

Pleural Effusion

Pleural effusion is rare in sarcoidosis and other causes such as cardiac disease should be considered before retaining the diagnosis (Figure 18). Clustering of nodules and micronodules beneath pleura may give the appearance of pleural thickening [9].

6. COMPLICATIONS ASSESSMENT

6.1. Fungal Colonization

Cavitary lesions and bullae may be colonized by Aspergillus with a fungal ball and adjacent pleural thickening [9, 20]. Fungal colonization is considered to be a pejorative factor in the evolution of sarcoidosis and occurs in almost 2% of cases, most frequently in fibrotic types [6, 7] (Figure 19).

6.2. Pulmonary Hypertension

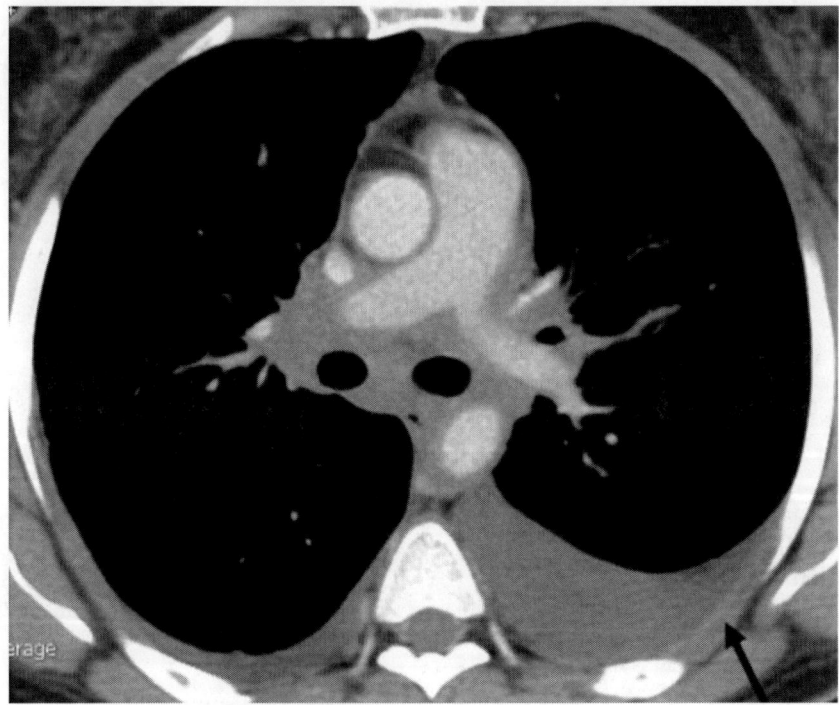

Figure 18. Pleural effusion with slight regular thickening of the pleura (arrow) and subcarinal as well as bilateral hilar lymph nodes.

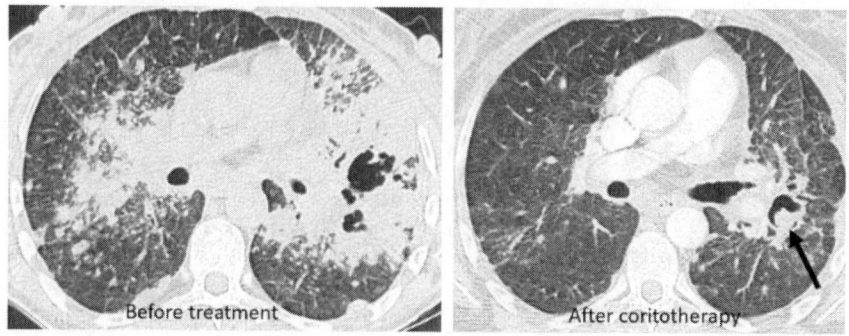

Figure 19. Fungal colonization in primary excavated sarcoïdosis undercorticotherapy (arrow).

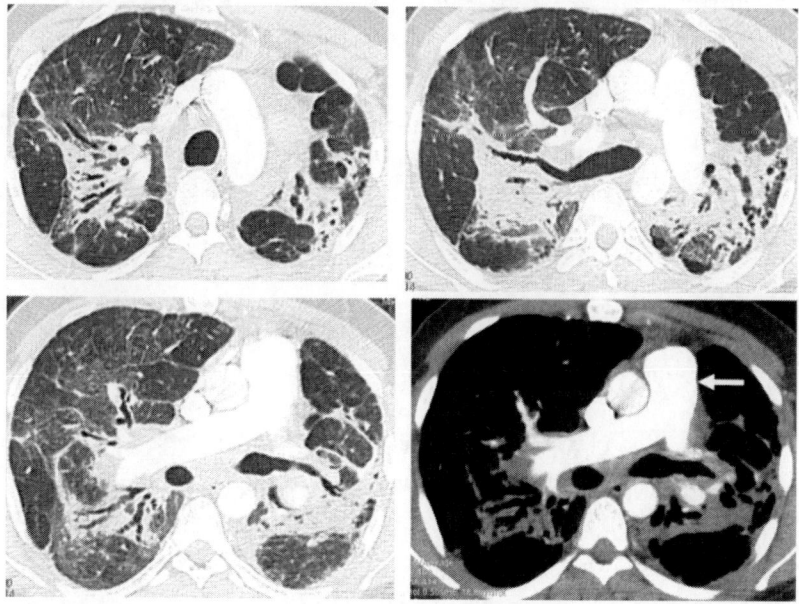

Figure 20. Fibrotic sarcoidosis with pulmonary trunk enlargement (arrow).

Pulmonary hypertension is a potential complication that is more common in type IV sarcoïdosis [20]. It occurs in 5 to 15% of patients and up to 50% in those who are symptomatic [9]. It can be explained by extrinsic compression of the central pulmonary vessels by lymphadenopathies or mediastinal fibrosis, granulomatous destruction of the pulmonary vessels, vasoreactivity, pulmonary veno-occlusive disease or sarcoid vasculopathy

[20, 21]. On CT, patients may have an enlargement of the main pulmonary trunk with a ratio of its diameter at the level of its bifurcation to the ascending aorta greater than 1 (Figure 20). Patients may also have right ventricle dilatation. Pulmonary hypertension is an independent pejorative prognostic factor in patients with severe disease with a 5-year survival rate of 60% [6].

CONCLUSION

Sarcoidosis is a multi-systemic disease in which lung involvement widely varies with typical and atypical active as well as fibrotic lesions. CT is a major imaging tool for diagnosis, especially in challenging cases. It makes it possible to follow up and detect complications.

REFERENCES

[1] Dubaniewicz, A. (2010). Mycobacterium tuberculosis heat shock proteins and autoimmunity in sarcoidosis. *Autoimmunity Reviews*, 9, 419-424.
[2] Van Enschot, J. W. T. & Van Balkom, R. H. H. (2013). Sarcoidosis following Mycobacterium tuberculosis infection: Coincidence or consequence. *Respiratory Medicine Case Reports*, 9, 11-14.
[3] Balan, A., Hoey, E. T. D., Sheerin, F., Lakkaraju, A. & Chowdhury, F. U. (2010). *Clinical Radiology*, 65, 750-760.
[4] Silva, M., Nunes, H., Valeyre, D. & Sverzellati, N. (2015). Imaging of Sarcoidosis. *Clinic Rev Allerg Immunol*, 49 (I), 45-53.
[5] Nunes, H., Uzunhan, Y., Gille, T., Lamberto, C., Valeyre, D. & Brillet, P. Y. (2015). *European Respir J*, 40, 750–765.
[6] Spagnolo, P., Sverzellati, N. & Wells, A. U. (2014). Hansell D. M. Imaging aspects of the diagnosis of sarcoidosis. *European Radiology*, 24 (IV), 807-16.

[7] Keijsers, R. G. M., Van den Heuvel, D. A. F. & Grutters, J. C. (2013). Imaging the inflammatory activity of sarcoidosis. *European Respir J*, *41*, 743–751.

[8] Nishinoa, M., Leea, K. S., Itohb, H. & Hatabu, H. (2010). The spectrum of pulmonary sarcoidosis: Variations of high-resolution CT findings and clues for specific diagnosis. *European Journal of Radiology*, *73*, 66–73.

[9] Iranmanesh, A. M. & Washington, L. (2018). Pulmonary Sarcoidosis: A Pictorial Review. *Seminars in Ultrasound CT and MRI*, doi: https://doi.org/10.1053/j.sult.2018.12.001.

[10] Brillet, P. Y., Nunesc, H., Soussana, M. & Brauner, M. W. (2011). Pulmonary sarcoidosis imaging. *Revue de Pneumologie Clinique*, *67*, 94—100.

[11] Little, B. P. (2015). Sarcoidosis: Overview of Pulmonary Manifestations andImaging. *Seminars in Roentgenology*, *50* (I), 52-64.

[12] Chiles, C. (2002). Imaging Features of Thoracic Sarcoidosis. *Seminars in Roentgenology*, *37* (I), 82-93.

[13] Salahuddin, M., Karanth, S., Ocazionez, D., Y-Martin, R. M. E. & Cherian, S. V. (2019). Clinical characteristics and etiologies of miliary nodules in the US; A single center study. *The American Journal of Medicine*. doi:https://doi.org/10.1016/j.amjmed. 2018.12. 030.

[14] Andreu, J., Mauleón, S., Pallisa, E., Majó, J., Martinez-Rodriguez, M. & Cáceres, J. (2002). Miliary Lung Disease Revisited. *Current Problems in Diagnostic Radiology*, *31*(V), 189-97.

[15] Hours, S., Nunes, H., Kambouchner, M., Uzunhan, Y., Brauner, M. W., Valeyre, D. & Brillet, P. Y. (2008). Pulmonary Cavitary Sarcoidosis - Clinico-Radiologic Characteristics and Natural History of a Rare Form of Sarcoidosis. *Medicine*, *87*, 142–151.

[16] Parkar, A. P. Kandiah. (2016). Differential Diagnosis of Cavitary Lung Lesions. *Journal of the Belgian Society of Radiology*, *100*(I), 100, 1–8.

[17] Handa, A., Dhooria, S., Sehgal, I. S. & Agarwal, R. (2018). Primary cavitary sarcoidosis: A case report, systematic review, and proposal of new diagnostic criteria. *Lung India*, *35*(I), 41–46.

[18] Margaritopoulos, G. A., Proklou, A., Lagoudaki, E., Voloudaki, A., Siafakas, N. M. & Antoniou, K. M. (2012). *Journal of Medical Case Reports*, *6*, 259-262.

[19] Trisolini, R., Anevlavis, S., Tinelli, C., Orlandi, P. & Patelli, M. (2013). CT pattern of lymphadenopathy in untreated patients undergoing bronchoscopy for suspected sarcoidosis. *Respiratory Medicine*, *107*, 897-903.

[20] Guidry, C., Fricke, R. G., Ram, R., Pandey, T. & Jambhekar, K. (2016). Imaging of Sarcoidosis: Contemporary Review. *Radiology Clinics of North America*, *54*(III), 519-34.

[21] Usunhan, Y. (2008). Sarcoïdose, les forms graves. *Revue des Maladies Respiratoires*, *25*, 77-78.

In: Interstitial Lung Disease
Editor: Liva T. Villadsen
ISBN: 978-1-53616-246-2
© 2019 Nova Science Publishers, Inc.

Chapter 5

CARDIO-PULMONARY TREATMENT IN SYSTEMIC SCLEROSIS PATIENTS: A CLINICAL GUIDE

Roberto G Carbone[1,], MD, Assaf Monselise[2], MD and Francesco Puppo[1], MD*

[1]Internal Medicine and Clinical Immunology Unit,
University of Genoa, Genoa, Italy
[2]Internal Medicine, private practice, Tel Aviv, Israel

ABSTRACT

About 10-15 percent of Systemic sclerosis (SSc) patients develop severe lung disease, which presents in two forms: a) pulmonary fibrosis (hardening or scarring of lung tissue because of collagen excess), b) pulmonary arterial hypertension (high blood pressure in the artery that carries blood from the heart to the lungs). Treatment for these two conditions is different. Pulmonary fibrosis may be treated with immunosuppressive drugs associated with low doses of corticosteroids, while pulmonary arterial hypertension (PAH) may be treated with drugs

---

* Corresponding Author's Email: carbone.roberto@aol.com.

that dilate blood vessels such as prostacyclin. In order to improve quality of life (QOL) and prognosis of SSc patients, early diagnosis of cardio-pulmonary complications and a proper therapeutic approach are required. Aims of this chapter are to: 1) identify diagnostic procedures for early diagnosis of cardio-pulmonary complications; 2) delineate a proper methodology to monitor complications; 3) define therapeutic guidelines.

Keywords: systemic sclerosis, interstitial lung diseases, pulmonary arterial hypertension, therapy, cardio- vascular complications, high resolution lung CT lung

GLOSSARY

6 MWT	6 minutes walk test
BAL	bronco- alveolar lavage
DLco	diffusion capacity of the lung for carbon monoxide
FVC	forced vital capacity
HRCT	high resolution computed tomography
ILD	interstitial lung disease
IPF	idiopathic pulmonary fibrosis
NSIP	non specific interstitial pneumonia
NYHA	New York Heart Association
PAH	pulmonary arterial hypertension
PAP	pulmonary artery pressure
PAPs	systolic pulmonary artery pressure
PAWP	pulmonary artery wedge pressure
PCWP	pulmonary capillary wedge pressure
PH	pulmonary hypertension
PVC	pulmonary vascular resistance
QOL	quality of life
SPECT	Single Photon Emission Computed Tomography
SSc	systemic sclerosis
Sv02	mixed venous oxygen saturation
UI	uptake index

UIP   usual interstitial pneumonia
WHO   World Health Organization.

1. INTRODUCTION

Systemic sclerosis (SSc) is a connective tissue disease involving several organs such as skin, esophagus, lungs, heart and kidneys [1]. Three pathological-mechanisms are involved in the pathogenesis of this disease: a) remodeling and thickening of vascular endothelium; b) early immune dys-regulation; c) fibroblast activation leading to excessive collagen deposition. It has been suggested that environmental factors interacting with a predisposing genetic background may lead to the development of this disease. Several mechanisms are involved with pulmonary complications: i) pulmonary alveolitis; ii) increased vascular resistances leading to early pulmonary arterial hypertension (PAH); iii) lung ventilatory damage. Interstitial lung disease (ILD) is the most important cause of mortality in patients suffering from SSc [1] and the correlation between ILD and PAH seems to be the major predictive cause of death [1, 2, 3, 4, 5].

1.1. Diagnostic Clinical Approach

Two different procedures are the gold standard in the diagnosis and monitoring of lung disease in SSc: high resolution computed tomography (HRCT) and ^{111}In-Octreotide scintigraphy (Octreoscan).

1.1.1. High Resolution CT

HRCT features of lung disease in patients with SSc closely resemble those seen in patients with non-specific idiopathic pneumonia (NSIP), which has recently been identified as the prevalent pattern found in lung biopsies. Nevertheless, HRCT features resembling idiopathic pulmonary fibrosis (IPF) with the presence of areas of honeycombing in combination with ground glass and reticular pattern at the bases of the lungs, which correspond on clinical examination with a bilateral "Velcro" sound, may be observed. Usually, in SSc patients areas of ground-glass pattern are greater than those observed in patients with Usual Interstitial Pneumonia (UIP) and are a reliable indicator of inflammation. Interestingly, in the clinical setting, a large extension of ground glass areas is predictive of better therapeutic response and good outcome.

With respect to the pathological pattern the numbers of fibroblastic foci, well-demarcated areas of proliferating fibroblasts, are a consistent finding in UIP. Enomoto et al. [6] showed that this scoring method of fibroblastic foci was more accurate than the semi-quantitative scoring methods in use. In fact, the number of such foci present in a lung biopsy is a good way for assessing disease activity and predicting poor prognosis of lung fibrosis in SSc [7] Several authors have established different severity scores of HRCT findings.[8, 9, 10] The presence of ground glass has been proved to be a valuable predictor both of response to therapy as well as of overall prognosis [11] In an early study, Wells et al. [9] found that the presence of ground glass opacity relative to findings of fibrosis was related to prognosis and likelihood of response to treatment In that study, HRCT abnormalities were interpreted as predominantly ground glass [9] (group 1), mixed ground glass opacity and reticular pattern (group 2), or opacities that were predominantly reticular pattern (group 3). In accordance with standard definitions such as those described by Wells et al. [9], and stressed by Lynch [12] we determined different HRCT patterns predicting prognosis. We grouped HRCT lung parenchyma abnormalities in four categories: Predominantly ground-glass pattern (level 1), ground glass and nodular cavities (level 2), mixed (ground glass and reticular pattern = level 3), or predominantly reticular pattern (level 4). For statistical reasons, in most of the analysis, levels have been re-grouped comparing levels 1 to 3 with the level 4. Two radiologists and two respiratory physicians met regularly and evaluated independently chest X-rays and HRCT findings in ILD patients. All patients with ILD underwent HRCT without intravenous contrast media and proceeding at 1,0 or 1,5 mm-thick sections taken at 1-cm intervals through the entire thorax.

1.1.2. Octreoscan: An Innovative Idea

Crestani et al. [13] showed that Octreoscan is an efficacious and accurate tool in monitoring IPF in SSc patients. Octreoscan, whole-body scans were obtained at 4 and 24-hours after administration of 5 mCi of [^{111}In-DTPA- D-Phe1]-Octreotide. Thoracic images were obtained with SPECT at the same intervals after injecting the tracer. Whole body acquisition (in 25 minutes) included anterior and posterior views of head, thorax, abdomen, pelvis and legs. Scintigraphic images were acquired with a double-head camera. The SPECT acquisition was performed with a double Indium photo-peak; slices were reconstructed after back projection, using a Butterworth (low pass) filter. Octreoscan U. I. defined as the ratio between normalised accumulation of the tracer in the lungs and thigh, was evaluated in correlation with the diagnosis, and conventional imaging. Normal values of U. I. on 4-h and 24-h were obtained. According to these data, the normal value of U. I. at 24-h was fixed at ≤10 U. I. [14]. Indium remains in the interstitium for a small period, and notably indium tracer can be useful for information regarding prognosis of lung fibrosis in SSc. Prognosis of lung fibrosis in SSc can be obtained by Octreoscan, and proposed as most promising tool in monitoring of this disease [13]. HRCT features of lung disease in patients with SSc closely resemble those of patients with NSIP - the typical histological pattern observed in SSc. Proportion of ground-glass opacity is greater in patients suffering from SSc than in patients with IPF - UIP.

Lebtahi et al. [15] described an increased Octreoscan U. I. in patients with SSc with respect to IPF. Carbone et al. [16] confirmed that Octreoscan U. I. is useful in differentiating IPF from NSIP, and in monitoring extra - thoracic sarcoidosis. This ancillary test could be a new and accurate method for identifying poor survival in IPF characterized by fibrosis, compared to NSIP and other interstitial lung diseases which are characterized by a considerable lymphocytic infiltrate.

1.1.3. Pulmonary Hypertension

PH is defined the mean of pulmonary arterial hypertension estimated by right cardiac catheterization, and normal value is > - 25 mm Hg [17]. In mass screening studies, echocardiography can be a valuable substitute for cardiac catheterization [18].

PAH is a serious complicating cause of mortality in SSc, especially when associated with ILD. Prevalence of PAH in limited scleroderma (CREST syndrome) by cardiac catheterize studies is 8% [19]. European Respiratory Society and European Cardiology Society guidelines recommend early diagnosis of PH by screening SSc patients [20]. Incidence of PAH among SSc patients is 15- 30% in large PH registries [21], while the prevalence of PAH is 5-12% [22]. In a French study PAH incidence was 0.6 per 100 cases, and PH (group 2) was the same range [21, 23]..

According to the WHO PH can be classified as pre- capillary isolated PAH (Group 1) or related to ILD described in Group 3 or post-capillary pulmonary hypertension included in Group 2 [20].

Few studies demonstrated the utility of 6- minutes walk test (6-MWT) and right atrial pressure as predictive of [24, 25], while other studies failed to confirm this or did not assess these variables [26, 27, and 28]. In add cardiac index in SSc has not been evaluated in some studies while others studies have confirmed this as a prognostic factor. All discrepancies can be explained why cardiac pulmonary pressure showed data discordant with respect to survival in SSc (i.e., right heart pressure and mean PAP).

A meta - analysis and a systematic review [5] included 2244 patients suffering from PH in combination with SSc. Results confirmed diffusion capacity of lung for carbon monoxide (DLco), NYHA, effusion pericardial, right atrial pressure, pulmonary vascular resistance (PVC), pulmonary artery wedge pressure (PAWP) cardiac index and mixed venous oxygen saturation (SvO2) and be poor significant anti-centromere antibody, forced vital capacity (FVC) and pulmonary capillary wedge pressure (PCWP) as accurate predictors of survival among these patients. [5].

A good correlation between gene profiles and PAH has been shown among SSc patients. Specifically, gene THB51 seems to be an important mediator in the development PAH predominant phenotype [29].

ILD is more common in diffuse cutaneous SSc (dsSSc) and often complicated by pulmonary hypertension [3]. Among these patients NSIP is the most common histologic pattern.

Cottin et al. [30] identified different risk factors related to ILD among SSc patients such as 1) dcSSc, 2) ethnicity, 3) older age at disease onset, 4) anti- Scl -70 anti- topo- isomerase I antibodies, and 5) absence of anticentromere antibody.

According to the EULAR Scleroderma Trials and Research Group (EUSTAR) database ILD was a cause of death among 35% of SSc patients during years 2004-2008 [31]. Similar data was collected from 2719 death certificates of SSc French patients in years 2000 and 2011 [32]. Indeed, half of death cases were due to cardiac –respiratory diseases and the percentage of deaths associated with SSc increased over this period [32].

Two histological subsets of NSIP - cellular and fibrotic NSIP - could help evaluate survival and outcome.

In our study (data non –published) we evaluated the clinical utility of indicators of survival in cellular and fibrotic patterns of NSIP among SSc patients. Twenty nine patients with NSIP were observed between January 1995 and December 2006: 11 patients with cellular NSIP and 18 patients with fibrotic NSIP. All patients underwent lung biopsy. Variables included in the analysis were: a) age at diagnosis b) smoking habits, c) New York Heart Association (NYHA) class, d) systolic Pulmonary Artery Pressure (PAPs), e) HRCT of lung, f) Octreoscan UI,, g) medications (prednisone alone or in combination with cyclofosfamide). Results showed that all patients with NSIP cellular pattern survived, while seven patients (64%) with fibrotic NSIP succumbed ($p = 0.0003$), median survival was 49 months. Age among NSIP patients was a prognostic indicator of survival ($p < 0.05$). Lung HRCT was a prognostic indicator of survival ($p < 0.05$). PAPs in NSIP was a strong and significant prognostic indicator of survival ($p < 0.01$) (Figure 1, 2, 3, 4.5, 6).

NYHA class in NSIP was a strong and significant prognostic indicator of survival ($p < 0.01$) Octreoscan UI was correlated with the histological findings in NSIP.

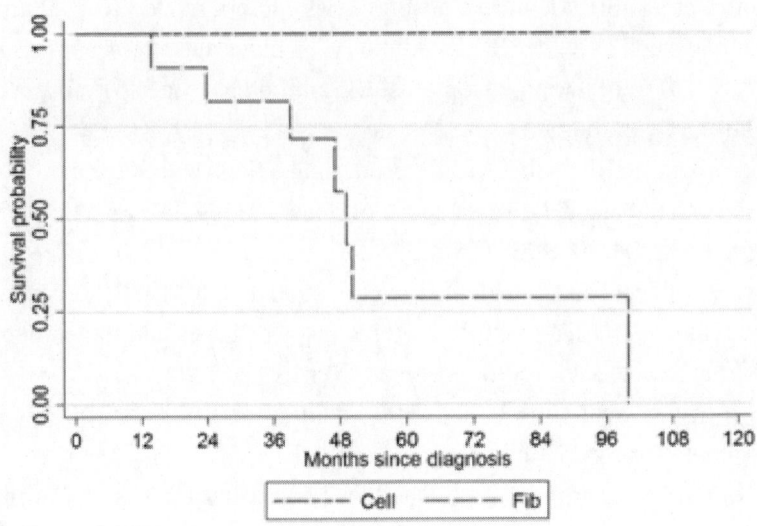

Figure 1. SSc -NSIP cellular and fibrotic subsets compared with survival. The graphic showed no patients with NSIP cellular patterns was deceased, conversely 7 patients (64%) with NSIP fibrotic was deceased (p = 0.0003). Median survival was 49 months.

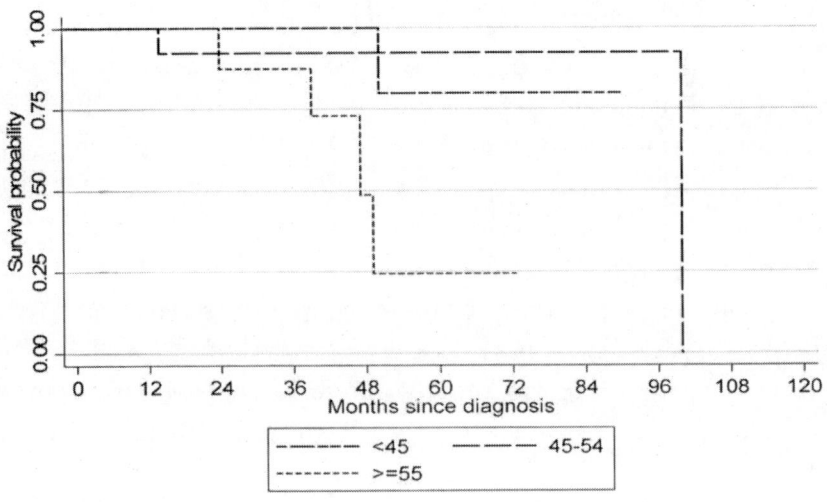

Figure 2. The graphic showed that in NSIP age was a statistical prognostic survival ($p < 0.05$).

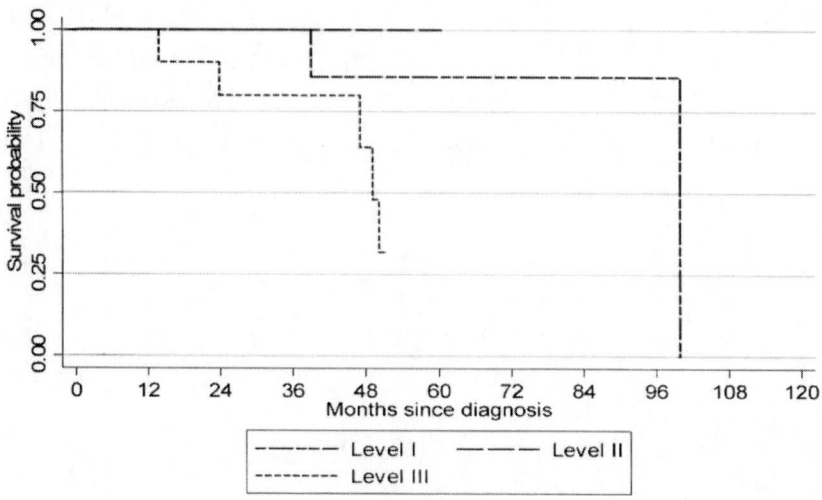

Figure 3. HRCT of lung was a statistical significant survival factor ($p < 0.05$).

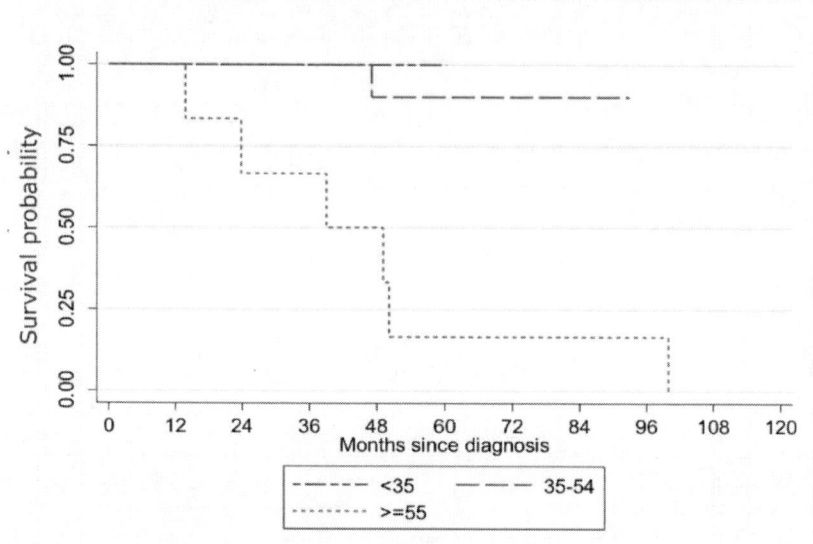

Figure 4. In NSIP, PAPs was strongly significant prognostic survival factor ($p < 0.01$).

The prospective evaluation of the study showed that 1) patients with a fibrotic NSIP pattern had a lower survival rate compared to those with the cellular pattern, 2) pulmonary hypertension identified by PAPs and NYHA class seems to be the best survival indicator and is stronger than age and lung HRCT.

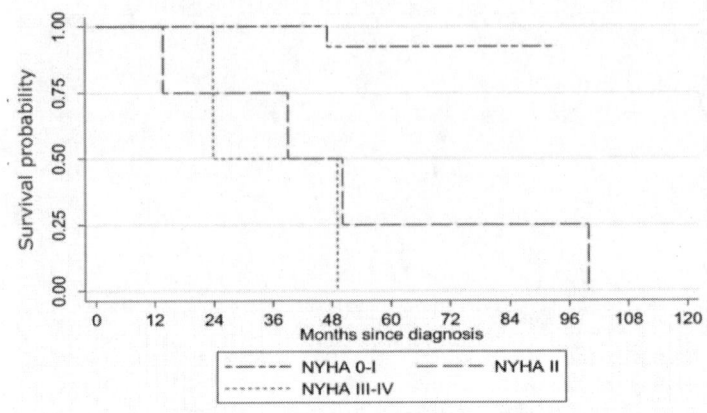

Figure 5. In NSIP New York Heart Association (NYHA) class was strongly significant prognostic survival factor ($p < 0.01$).

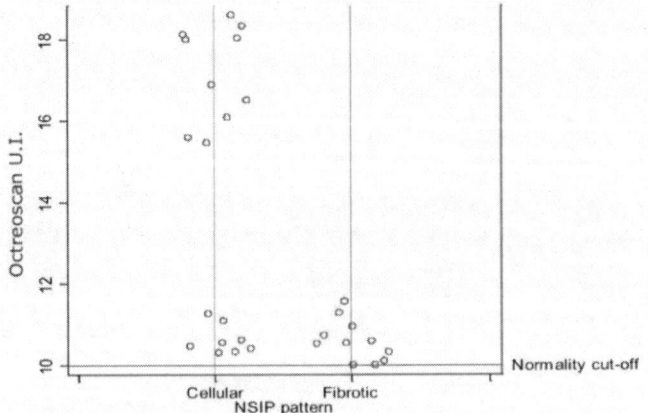

Figure 6. The graphic depicted in NSIP Octreoscan uptake index (U: I.) with correlated with histological findings.

To illustrate our results series of lung HRCT's of in NSIP and histology findings are herein reported (Figure 7, 8, 9, 10, 11, 12 13, 14).

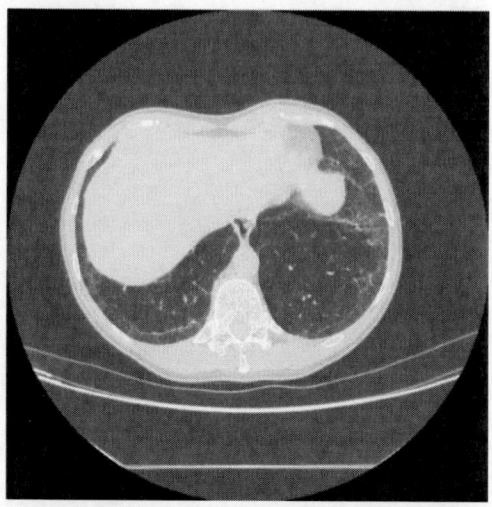

Figure 7. HRCT of lung in early diagnosis of SSc – NISP showed on the left of the lung typical ground glass opacities.

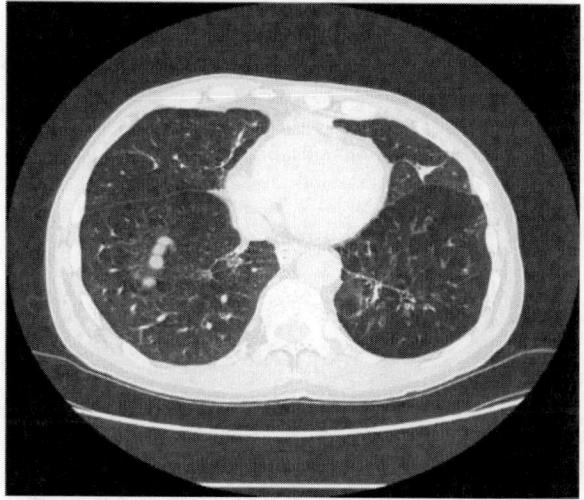

Figure 8. HRCT of lung showed a combination of obstructive and restrictive patterns as NSIP fibrotic and emphysema on the left of the lung.

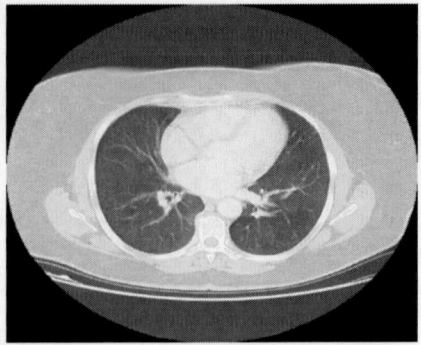

Figure 9. An early diagnosis of SSc-NSIP histological cellular pattern was reported here on HRCT of the lung. In detail on the left of the lung.

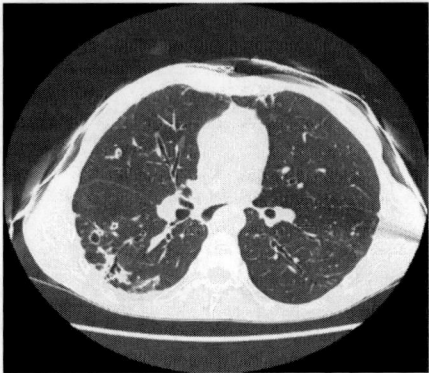

Figure 10. HRCT of lung revealed a bilateral SSc -NSIP mixed patterns on the basis of the lungs where were present a reticular and ground glass pattern.

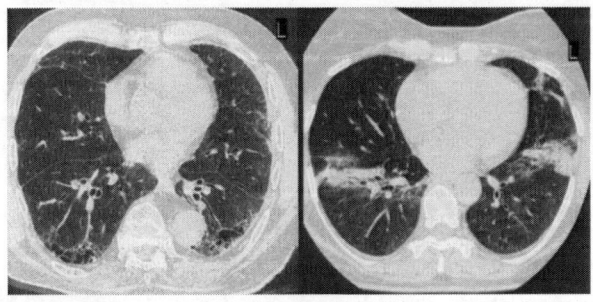

Figure 11. HRCT on the left showed a typical SSc –IPF with honeycombing pattern on the basis of bilateral lungs compared with advanced SSc-NSIP patterns present n HRCT on the right. Notably the latter showed several areas of ground glass opacities evident on bilateral lungs.

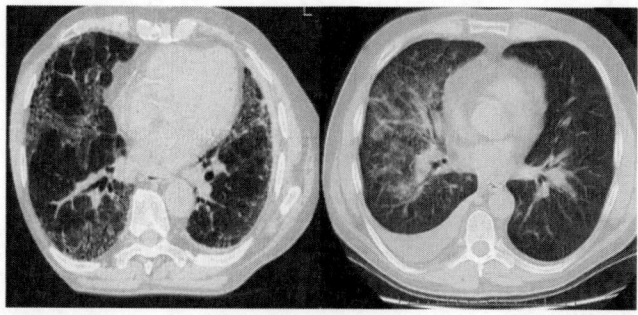

Figure 12. On the left the picture of HRCT showed SSc - NSIP pattern compared with an advanced fibrotic pattern of sarcoidosis HRCT.

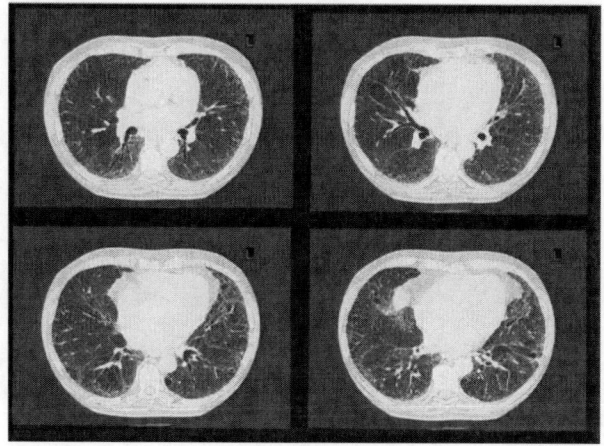

Figure 13. An advanced lung involvement in fatal typical SSc –IPF pattern with honeycombing present in all HRCT figures.

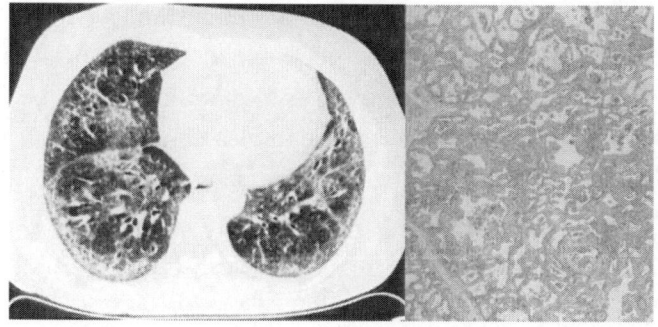

Figure 14. A comparison between HRCT SSc-typical advanced IPF pattern confirmed by a histological compromised findings.

An additional risk factor in SSc is pulmonary embolism, when antiphospholipids antibodies are present [33, 34, 35].

1.1.4. Monitoring and Outcome

Table 1. Flow diagram for the clinical assessment of Systemic Sclerosis

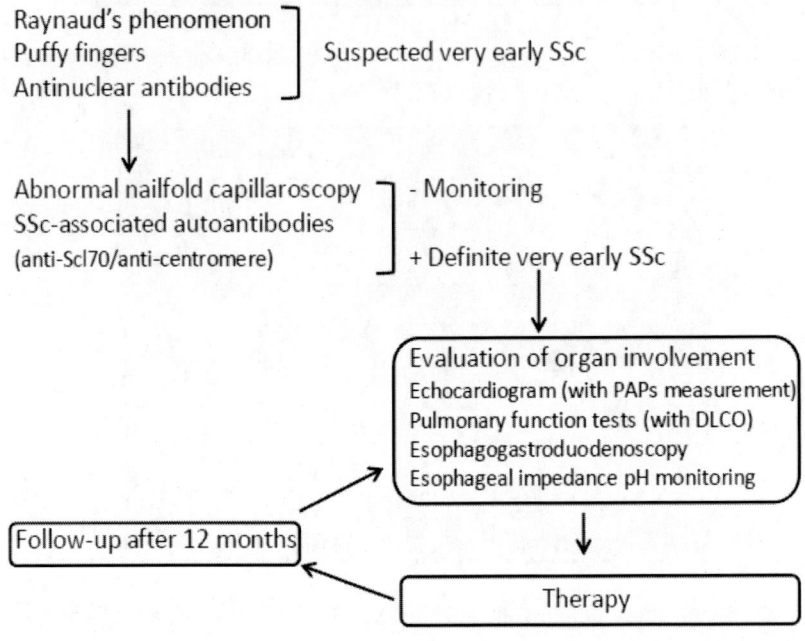

When monitoring SSc patients the preferred method would be an index that expresses patients' well being such as: a) Quality of Life (QOL), symptoms (dyspnea and cough) as well as b) mortality rate and, c) the time to disease development. Using a flow-chart as a clinical guide (Table 1) in screening populations, applying correct diagnostic procedures, and identifying the cut-off of disease severity during follow–up, (Table 2a) [36, 37, 38, 39, 40, 41, 42, 43, 44, 45], (Table 2b) [46], monitoring patients at baseline, 6-months, and one yearly after, (Table 3) Indeed co-morbidities may be avoided by early treatment, thereby reducing treatment costs.

Table 2a. Severity disease score in Systemic Sclerosis patients with cardio – pulmonary complications

Cough Score°	FVC ^	DLCO ^	HRCT score *	NYHA**	PAPS **	QOL***	Grade severity§
0	≥80%	≥80%	<2	0	<35	0	0
1	70-79%	70-79%	≥2	1	35–55	1	1
2	50-79%	50-79%	3	2	>55	2	2
3	<50%	<50%	4	3	RV↓↓ function	3	3
4	<50%	<50%	5	4	RV↓↓↓	3	4

Source: Severity level calculated according to Petty TL et al. [36]. ^ In agreement with ATS standard parameters [37-38].*Visual score adopted and reported by Kazeeroni et al. [39]. **Estimated values in agreement with Olschewski et al. [40]. ***Severity score calculated in agreement with Steen VD et al. [41], and with Clements et al. [42]. §Octreoscan uptake index (UI) score [44,45].

Table 2b. Modified Rodnan skin Score

17 surface anatomic areas of the body

Face
Anterior chest
Abdomen
Fingers   (right and left)
Forearms   (right and left)
Upper arms   (right and left)
Tights   (right and left)
Lower legs   (right and left)
Dorsum of hands   (right and left)
Dorsum of feet   (right and left)

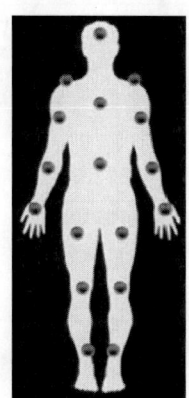

These individual values are added and the sum is defined as the total skin score (Maximum 51)

Note: The score consists of an evaluation of patient's skin thickness rated by clinical palpation: 0 = normal skin; 1 = mild thickness; 2 = moderate thickness; 3 = severe thickness with inability to pinch the skin into a fold [46].

Table 3. Flow-chart. Clinical diagnostic examination and follow-up in Systemic Sclerosis

Variables	Baseline	Follow-up 6 months	Follow- up 12 months
Age	•		
Gender	•		
Smoking/habits	•	•	•
Cough – score	•	•	•
Clinical exam	•	•	•
Chest x ray	•		
Cardiogram	•		
Echocardiography	•		•
Co-morbidity	•		•
CRP	•	•	•
Auto-antibody	•		•
Spirometry (FVC – DLCO)	•	•	•
Arterial blood test	•	•	•
Rodnan skin test	•	•	•
Plicometry	•	•	•
Body Mass Index	•	•	•
6-MWT	•	•	•
NYHA class	•	•	•
PAPS	•		•
HRCT lung-score	•		•
QOL	•	•	•
BAL	•		•
Octreoscan (U.I.)	•		•

1.1.5. Formula

$$\frac{\text{Patient's numbers with Systemic sclerosis and pulmonary complications}}{\text{Patient's numbers with Systemic sclerosis without pulmonary complications}}$$

1.1.6. Variables

At baseline two variables for monitoring are highlighted: a) SSc subjects with pulmonary complications, QOL, and outcome at 6 –months and at one year. from baseline and identifying as well SSc subjects without pulmonary complications, and verifying the risk of disease and how long they can arise, b) Clinical assessment of subjects related to possible complications, and evaluating the improvement of QOL during the period monitored correlated to a decrease of treatment and a reduction of costs as well.

1.1.7. Data Analysis

Variables at baseline follow up at 6 and 12 months respectively, (Table 3) needs about the outcome examined. Octreoscan (normal value of uptake index was ≤10, [40].

1.1.8. Treatment of Systemic Sclerosis Associated Pulmonary Arterial Hypertension

Several drugs have been studied and approved for use in patients with systemic sclerosis related pulmonary arterial hypertension (SSc-PAH). Drug use and treatment regimens for SSc-PAH patients have been recently extensively reviewed [47, 48] and will be briefly discussed in the present section.

The endothelin receptor antagonists (ERA) bosentan, ambrisentan and macitentan have been shown to improve exercise tolerance and hemodynamics in SSc-PAH patients. Bosentan is an oral dual ERA (62.5 mg twice daily, then if tolerated 125 mg twice daily), which blocks both type A (ETA) and type B (ETB) receptors. Ambrisentan is an oral ERA (taken at a dose of 5 mg once daily, then increased as needed and tolerated to a maximum of 10 mg once daily) with elevated specificity for the ETA receptor. Macitentan is an oral ETA and ETB receptor antagonist (10 mg once daily) that leads to reduced mortality in patients with PAH-SSc. Adverse events associated with ERA treatment include abnormal liver function tests, peripheral oedema, palpitations, headache, chest pain, nasal congestion and anaemia.

The phosphodiesterase 5 (PDE-5) inhibitors sildenafil (20 mg three times daily) and tadalafil (40 mg once daily) are oral medications which result in vasodilatation. They improve exercise tolerance, functional status and quality of life and reduce clinical worsening. Side effects associated with PDE-5 inhibitors include flushing, dyspepsia, diarrhoea, headache and myalgia.

The guanylate cyclase stimulator (GCs) riociguat is given orally (from 0.5–2.5 mg three times daily). It has been shown to improve 6MWT, WHO functional class and hemodynamic parameters. Several serious adverse events including syncope, increase in hepatic enzyme levels, dizziness, acute renal failure and hypotension have been reported after riociguat intake.

Prostacyclins, i.e., epoprostenol, iloprost, and treprostinil, are potent vasodilators with additional antiproliferative and antiplatelet effects. Prostacyclins ameliorate exercise tolerance, dyspnea and functional class. Epoprostenol is given in an appropriated clinical setting by continuous I. V. infusion through a central venous catheter. Epoprostenol may incite severe adverse events (infections, pneumothorax and haemorrhage) and several side effects (headache, jaw pain, diarrhoea, abdominal pain, anorexia, vomiting, photosensitivity, and cutaneous flushing). Iloprost is available as inhaled (in USA) and intravenous (in EU) formulations and treprostinil is available as subcutaneous or intravenous infusion as well as inhaled and oral forms. Iloprost and treprostinil dose depends on the administration route and individual tolerance. Iloprost infusion can commonly induce headache, flushing, nausea and sweat. Side effects associated with usage of intravenous treprostinil are similar to that reported with intravenous epoprostenol, subcutaneous treprostinil injection may be associated with pain at the infusion site. Inhaled prostanoids use can result in cough, headache, flushing, nausea and syncope. Selexipag is an oral prostacyclin receptor agonist (starting dose of 200 mcg twice daily, then increased by 200 mcg twice daily every week to the highest tolerated dose up to a maximum of 1,600 mcg twice daily) that has been shown to delay reduction in functional capacity.

Several studies showed improved outcomes and better survival for SSc-PAH patients with combination therapy (i.e., ambrisentan and tadalafil or ERA and PDE-5 inhibitors) compared to either therapy alone.

The treatment of co-morbidities (heart failure, Obstructive Sleep Apnea Syndrome, hypertension) is warranted in order to ameliorate prognosis. Concurrent medications use (calcium channel blockers, beta blockers, nitrates) may be taken also into account. Anticoagulation of SSc-PAH patients is a controversial issue and further studies are necessary.

Based on the results of randomised controlled trials, the European League against Rheumatism (EULAR) recommends intravenous epoprostenol for the treatment of patients with severe SSc-PAH class III and IV (strength of recommendation A) and ERA, PDE-5 inhibitors, prostacyclin analogues and riociguat to treat less severe SSc-PAH (strength of recommendation B) [49]. In severe selected cases of SSc-PAH lung transplantation may be proposed.

Ongoing trials are currently evaluating the potential efficacy of elastase inhibitor (Elastin) and anti-CD20 monoclonal antibody (Rituximab) in SSc-PAH patients.

Proposed step-up regimens for the treatment of SSc-PAH

6MWT (m)*	WHO Functional Class	TREATMENT**
600	I	Monotherapy (PDE-5 inhibitor/ERA/GCs/prostacyclin)
400	II	PDE-5 inhibitor + ERA
300	III	PDE-5 inhibitor + ERA + Inhaled or oral prostacyclin
150	IV	PDE-5 inhibitor + ERA + Parenteral prostacyclin

*6-Minute-Walking Test, ** for abbreviations see text.

CONFLICTS OF INTEREST

The Authors do not have conflicts of interest.

REFERENCES

[1] LeRoy, E. C., Black, C., Fleischmajer, R., et al. Scleroderma (systemic sclerosis) classification, subsets and pathogenesis. *J Rheumatol* 1988; 15; 202-5.

[2] White, B., Moore, W. C., Wigley, F. M., et al. Cyclofosphamide is associated with pulmonary function and survival benefit in patients with scleroderma and alveolitis. *Ann Intern Med* 2000; 132: 947-954.

[3] Trad, S., Zahir, A., Beigelman, C, et al. Pulmonary arterial hypertension is a major mortality factor in diffuse systemic sclerosis, independent of interstitial lung disease. *Arthritis & Rheumatism* 2006; 54:184-191.

[4] Mathai, S., Hunmers, L. K., Champion, H. C. et al. Survival in pulmonary hypertension associated with the scleroderma spectrum of diseases. *Arthritis & Rheumatism* 2009; 60 (2): 569-577.

[5] Lefevre G, Dauchet L, Hachulla e, et al. survival and prognostic factors in systemic sclerosis associated pulmonary hypertension. *Arthritis & Rheumatism* 2013; 65 (5) 2412-2423.

[6] Enomoto, N., Suda, T., Kato, M., et al. Quantitative analysis of fibroblastic foci in usual interstitial pneumonia. *Chest.* 2006 Jul;130 (1)3-5.

[7] Titto, L., Bloigu, R., Heiskanen, U. et al. Relationship between hystopathological features and the course of idiopathic pulmonary fibrosis/usual interstitial pneumonia. *Thorax* 2006; 61:1091-95.

[8] Zompatori, M., Fasano, L., Rimondi, M. R., et al. The assessment of the activity of idiopathic pulmonary fibrosis by high-resolution computed tomography. *Radiol Med 1996*; 91(3):238-46.

[9] Wells, A. U., Hansell, D. M., Rubens, M. B., et al. The predictive value of appearances on thin-section computed tomography in fibrosing alveolitis. *Am Rev Respir Dis.* 1993; 148:1076-82.

[10] MacDonald, S. L., Rubens, M. B., Hansell, D. M., et al. Non specific interstitial pneumonia and usual interstitial pneumonia: comparative appearances at and diagnostic accuracy of thin-section CT. *Radiology.* 2001; 221(3):583-4.

[11] High-resolution CT of the lung. Webb, R., Müller, N., Naidich, D. Eds. Lippincott Williams & Wilkins, Philadelphia (USA) 2001.
[12] Lynch, D. A. Non specific interstitial pneumonia. Evolving concepts. *Radiology* 2001: 221: 583-584.
[13] Crestani, B. J., Chapron, B., Wallaert, E. et al. Octreotide treatment of idiopathic pulmonary fibrosis: a proof-of-concept study *European Respiratory Journal* 2012 39: 772-775.
[14] Carbone, R., Filiberti, R., Grosso, M., et al. Octreoscan perspectives in sarcoidosis and idiopathic interstitial pneumonia. *Eur Rev Med Pharmacol Sci.* 2003 Jul-Aug;7(4):97-105.
[15] Lebtahi, R., Moreau, S., Marchand-Adam, S. et al. Increased uptake of ^{111}In-octreotide in idiopathic pulmonary fibrosis. *J Nucl Med.* 2006 Aug; 47(8):1281-7.
[16] Carbone, R. Bottino, G., Paredi, P. et al, Predictors of survival in idiopathic interstitial pneumonia *European Review for Medical and Pharmacological Sciences* 2010; 14: 695-704.
[17] McGoon, M. D., Benza, R. L., Escribamos Subias et al. Pulmonary arterial hypertension epidemiology and registries. *J Am Coll Cardiol* 2013; 62: 25 Suppl. D51: D59.
[18] McGoon, M., Gutterman, D., Steen, V. et al. Screening early detection and diagnosis of pulmonary arterial hypertension ACCP evidence based clinical practice guidelines. *Chest 2004*; 126: 14S:34S.
[19] Lynch, D. A. Lung disease related to collagen vascular disease. *J Thorac Imaging* 2009; 24 (4) 299: 309.
[20] Galie' N, Humbert M, Vachery JL et al. ESC-ERS guidelines for the diagnosis and treatment of pulmonary hypertension: the joint task force for the diagnosis and treatment of pulmonary hypertension of the European Society of Cardiology (ESC) and European Respiratory Society (ERS). Enclosed by Association European Paediatric and Congenital Cardiology (AEPC), International Society for Heart and Lung Transplantation (ISHLT)- *Eur Heart J* 2016; 3767- 119.
[21] Avouac J, Airo P, Meune C et al. Prevalence of pulmonary hypertension in sysstemic sclerosis in European Caucasian systemic meta-analysis of 5 studies. *J Rheumatol* 2010; 37: 2290- 2298.

[22] Hachulla E, de Groote T, Gressin V et al. The three-year incidence of pulmonary arterial hypertension associated with systemic sclerosis in a multicenter nationwide longitudinal study in France. *Arthritis Rheum* 2009; 60: 1831-1839.
[23] Simonneau G, Gatzoulis MA, Adatia A et al. Update Clinical Classification of pulmonary hypertension. *J Am Coll Cardiol* 2013; 62 D 34-41.
[24] Condliffe R, Kiely DG, Peacock AJ, et al. Connective tissue disease-associated pulmonary arterial hypertension in the modern treatment era. *Am Respir Crit Care Med* 2009; 79: 151-7.
[25] Williams MH, Handler CE, Akram R, et al. Role of N-terminal natriuretic peptide (N-TproBNP) in scleroderma-associated pulmonary arterial hypertension. *Eur Heart J* 2006; 1485-94.
[26] Humbert M, Berezne A, et al. Clinical characteristics and survival in systemic sclerosis-related pulmonary hypertension associated with interstitial lung disease. *Chest* 2011; 140: 1016-24.
[27] Campo A, Mathai SC, Le Pavec J et al. Hemodynamic predictors of survival in scleroderma related pulmonary arterial hypertension. *Am J Respir Crit Care Med* 2010:182: 252-60.
[28] Launay D, Sitbon O, Cordier JF et al. Survival and prognosis factors in patients incident and newly diagnosed SSc- associated pulmonary arterial hypertension from the French Registry. *Am Rheum Dis*, in press.
[29] Moll M, Christmann RB, Zhang Y, et al. Patients with systemic-sclerosis –associated pulmonary arterial hypertension express a genomic signature distinct from patients with interstitial lung disease. *J Scleroderma Relat Disord* 2018; 3 (3) 242-248.
[30] Cottin V, KK Brown. Interstitial lung disease associated with systemic sclerosis (SSc –ILD). *Respiratory Research* 2019; 20: (13) 1-10.
[31] Tyndall A, Banner B, Vonk M et al. Cause and risk factors to death in systemic sclerosis a study for the EULAR scleroderma trial and research (EUSTAR) database. *Ann Rheum Dis* 2010; 69(10):809-15.
[32] Elhai M, Meune C, Boubaya M, et al. Mapping and predicting mortality from systemic sclerosis. *Ann Rheum Dis* 2017; 76: 897-905.

[33] Schoenfeld, S. R., Choi, H. K., Sayre, E. C. et al. Risk of pulmonary embolism and deep venous thmbosis in systemic sclerosis: a general population based study. *Arthritis Care Res* 2016; 68: 246-253.

[34] Ungprasert, P., Srivali, N., Kittanamongkolchai, W. Systemic sclerosis and risk of venous thromboembolism: a systemic review and meta-analysis. *Mod Rheumatol* 2015; 25: 893-897.

[35] Chung, W. S., Lin, C. I., Sung, F. C. et al. Systemic sclerosis increases the risks of deep vein thrombosis and pulmonary thomboembolism: a nationwide cohort study. *Rheumatology* 2014; 53: 1639-1645.

[36] Petty, T. L. The National Mucolytic Study. Results of a randomised double-blind, placebo-controlled study of iodinated glycerol in chronic obstructive bronchitis. *Chest* 1990; 98: 75-83.

[37] American Thoracic Society. Standardization of Spirometry – 1994 Uptdate. *Am J Respir Crit Care Med* 1995. 152:1107-36.

[38] American Thoracic Society. Single breath carbon monoxide diffusing capacity (transfer factor). Recommendation for a standard technique 1995 Update. *Am J Respir Crit Care Med* 1995. 152:2185-98.

[39] Kazerooni, E. A., Martinez, F. J., Flint, A., et al. Thin – section CT at 10 mm increments versus limited three-level thin-section CT for idiopathic pulmonary fibrosis: Correlation with pathologic scoring. *AJR Am J Roentgenol* 1997; 169: 977-983.

[40] Olschewski, H., Seeger, W., Olschewski, S. *Pulmonary hypertension: Pathophysiology, Diagnosis, Treatment, and Development.* UNI-MED SCIENCE ed. 2002. Bremen, Germany.

[41] Steen, V. D., Medsger Jr., T. A. The value of the Health Assessment Questionnaire and special patient-generated scales to demonstrate change in systemic sclerosis patients over time. *Arthritis & Rheum* 1997; 40: 1984-1991.

[42] Clements, P. J., Wong, W. K., Hurwitz, E. L., et al. The disability index of the Health Assessment Questionnaire is a predictor and correlate of outcome in high-dose vs. low-dose penicillamine in systemic sclerosis trial. *Arthritis & Rheum* 2001; 44: 653-661.

[43] ATS Statement: Guidelines for the Six-Minute Walk Test. *Am J Respir crit. Care Med.* 2002; 166: 111-117.

[44] Carbone, R. G., Monselise, A., Bottino, G. Pulmonary hyper tension in interstitial lung disease. In: Baughman RP, Carbone RG, Bottino G. (eds.) *Pulmonary Arterial Hypertension and Interstitial Lung Diseases*. New York: Springer 2009;pp. 13-50.

[45] Carbone, R., Balleari, E., Grosso, M., et al. Predictors of mortality of idiopathic pulmonary fibrosis. *Eur Rev Med Pharmacol Sci* 2008; 12: 97-104.

[46] Clements, P. J., Lachenbruch, P. A., Seibold, J. R., et al. Skin thickness score in systemic sclerosis: an assessment of interobserver variability in 3 independent studies. *J Rheumatol.* 1993; 20:1892–6.

[47] Sundaram, S. M. & Chung, L. An update on Systemic Sclerosis-associated pulmonary arterial hypertension: a review of the current literature. *Curr Rheum Rep* 2018; 20: 1-10.

[48] Denton C. P., Wells A. U., Coghlan J. G. Major lung complications of systemic sclerosis. *Nat Rev Rheumatol* 2018; 14: 511-527.

[49] Kowal-Bielecka O., et al. Update of EULAR recommendations for the treatment of systemic sclerosis. *Ann Rheum Dis* 2017; 76: 1327–1339.

INDEX

A

Acute Eosinophilic Pneumonia (AEP), vii, viii, 76, 77, 84, 85, 94, 97, 98, 99, 104, 106, 107, 108
Acute Immunoallergic Pneumonia (AIAP), 77, 83, 97, 106
Acute infiltrative lung disease (AILD), v, viii, ix, 75, 76, 77, 78, 85, 86, 88, 91, 93, 94, 96, 97, 98, 99, 103, 104, 105, 106
Acute Organizing Pneumonia (AOP), 77, 81, 82, 93, 98, 99
air-trapping, 153
alveolar hemorrhage, ix, 76, 77, 78, 79, 80, 81, 82, 94, 95, 97, 99, 108, 111
amiodarone, 97, 98
ARDS, 78, 99, 102

B

bronchial distortion, x, 78, 124, 142, 146, 147, 148
bronchovascular bundle thickening, 102, 144

C

cardio- vascular complications, 162
cocaine, ix, 76, 81, 98, 110
computed tomography, 76, 101, 107, 117, 118, 119, 131, 138, 142, 143, 152, 162, 163, 180
connective tissue diseases, 47, 81, 93, 94, 105, 114, 115, 135
crazy paving, 79, 84, 86, 87, 95, 105, 106
cysts, 15, 86, 88, 121, 131, 132, 134
cytomegalovirus (CMV), 85, 88, 89, 91, 105

D

dermatopolymyositis, 93
diffuse acute infiltrative lung disease, 76
Diffuse Alveolar Damage (DAD), vii, viii, 76, 77, 78, 80, 84, 93, 94, 97, 98, 99, 101, 102, 103, 110, 119
Diffuse Alveolar Hemorrhage (DAH), vii, viii, 76, 77, 79, 81, 94, 95, 96, 98, 105, 106

Index

E

Eosinophilic Granulomatosis with Polyangiitis, 84, 94
eosinophilic pneumonia, ix, 76, 77, 84, 98

F

familial pulmonary fibrosis, 2, 6, 31, 50, 51, 54, 66, 67, 72
fibrosis, vii, viii, xi, 1, 2, 3, 4, 7, 10, 11, 13, 14, 15, 17, 23, 25, 26, 28, 29, 30, 31, 32, 33, 35, 36, 38, 39, 40, 47, 48, 49, 50, 51, 52, 54, 55, 56, 57, 59, 62, 63, 65, 66, 68, 69, 71, 72, 74, 78, 83, 100, 108, 115, 116, 119, 121, 122, 123, 124, 128, 129, 130, 132, 133, 136, 137, 139, 142, 143, 144, 146, 151, 157, 161, 164, 165
fibrotic forms, x, 142, 146, 151

G

GGO, 77, 78, 79, 82, 83, 84, 86, 89, 92, 97, 99, 100, 102, 105, 106, 116, 118, 127
Goodpasture Syndrome, 96
Granulomatosis with polyangiitis, 94
Ground glass opacities, 116, 151

H

Hamman-Rich syndrome, 49, 101
heroin, ix, 76, 98
HIA, 93, 98
high resolution lung CT lung, 162
High-resolution computed tomography (HR-CT), vii, x, 54, 92, 99, 102, 109, 114, 124, 135, 136, 139, 142, 143, 180
honeycombing, x, 17, 102, 115, 116, 117, 119, 120, 121, 122, 131, 133, 142, 146, 147, 148, 163, 172, 173

I

idiopathic pulmonary fibrosis, viii, 1, 2, 47, 49, 50, 51, 52, 53, 54, 57, 58, 59, 60, 61, 62, 63, 64, 65, 66, 67, 68, 70, 71, 72, 73, 99, 100, 102, 107, 109, 110, 111, 114, 136, 146, 162, 163, 180, 181, 183, 184
inflammation, vii, viii, 1, 2, 19, 22, 42, 48, 84, 115, 121, 122, 142, 143, 164
inflammatory active forms, x, 142
influenza, 85, 88, 90, 105
interstitial lung diseases, vii, viii, 1, 46, 47, 58, 74, 100, 136, 137, 139, 162, 165
irradiation, 99, 143
irregular linear pattern, x, 142, 146

L

Legionellosis, 92
Lesional pulmonary edema, 93, 99
leukostasis, 103
lung, vii, viii, ix, x, xi, 2, 5, 7, 10, 11, 12, 14, 15, 17, 19, 20, 27, 30, 35, 37, 38, 39, 40, 41, 42, 44, 47, 48, 50, 51, 52, 53, 54, 56, 57, 58, 61, 63, 65, 66, 68, 69, 70, 72, 73, 74, 75, 76, 80, 81, 83, 84, 85, 86, 87, 88, 98, 99, 100, 101, 102, 105, 106, 107, 108, 109, 110, 111, 113, 114, 115, 116, 118, 119, 120, 121, 122, 125, 126, 127, 128, 131, 134, 135, 138, 139, 142, 143, 148, 150, 151, 158, 161, 162, 163, 164, 165, 166, 167, 169, 170, 171, 172, 173, 176, 179, 180, 181, 182, 184
lymphangitic carcinomatosis, 103
lymphoma, 103, 134, 144

M

Macronodules, 149, 150
microscopic polyangiitis, 81, 94, 95, 106

miliary, x, 89, 91, 142, 148, 149, 159
mixed connective tissue disease, 93, 124
mucin, 2, 5, 13, 14, 57, 58
Mycobacteria, 85, 89, 91
Mycoplasma Pneumoniae, 88, 89

N

Non-Specific Interstitial Pneumonia, 15, 121, 128

O

Octreoscan, 163, 165, 167, 170, 175, 176, 177, 181

P

perilymphatic micronodules, 144
Pneumocystosis, 85, 86, 87, 88, 105
Propylthiouracil, 97
pseudo-masses, x, 142, 146
pulmonary arterial hypertension, xi, 161, 162, 163, 165, 177, 180, 181, 182, 184
Pulmonary Cardiogenic Edema, 92
Pulmonary cysts, 86, 87
Pulmonary Hypertension, 100, 156, 162, 165, 166, 170, 180, 181, 182

R

respiratory failure, 76, 89, 99, 101

S

sarcoidosis, v, vii, x, 15, 32, 57, 103, 119, 135, 141, 142, 143, 148, 151, 152, 153, 155, 156, 157, 158, 159, 160, 165, 173, 181
surfactant, 2, 8, 11, 12, 44, 50, 51, 52, 53, 54, 55, 56
systemic lupus erythematosu, 41, 81, 93, 128
systemic sclerosis, xi, 15, 46, 57, 124, 161, 162, 163, 177, 180, 182, 183, 184

T

telomerase, 2, 4, 24, 25, 26, 27, 29, 30, 31, 34, 35, 37, 38, 41, 44, 51, 64, 65, 66, 67, 68, 69, 70, 71
telomere, 2, 4, 7, 24, 25, 27, 29, 30, 31, 32, 33, 35, 36, 37, 38, 39, 40, 42, 43, 44, 50, 64, 65, 66, 67, 69, 70, 71, 72
therapy, 3, 18, 36, 38, 43, 111, 124, 125, 128, 162, 164, 178
TOLLIP, 2, 5, 6, 18, 40, 42, 59

V

vanishing lung syndrome, 151
Vasculitis, ix, 76, 77, 81, 94, 97, 105
Viruses, ix, 76, 85, 88, 105

Related Nova Publications

ACUTE LUNG INJURY: EPIDEMIOLOGY, HEALTH EFFECTS AND THERAPEUTIC TREATMENT STRATEGIES

EDITOR: Daniela Mokrá, MD, PhD

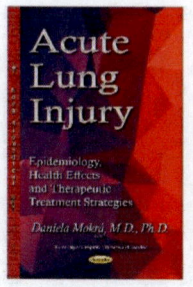

SERIES: Pulmonary and Respiratory Diseases and Disorders

BOOK DESCRIPTION: In this book, authors review the current knowledge on acute lung injury (ALI). ALI/acute respiratory distress syndrome (ARDS) is characterized by diffuse alveolar damage, alveolar capillary leakage, lung edema, neutrophil-derived inflammation, and surfactant dysfunction.

SOFTCOVER ISBN: 978-1-61470-426-3
RETAIL PRICE: $69

CYSTIC AND IDIOPATHIC PULMONARY FIBROSIS: RISK FACTORS, MANAGEMENT AND LONG-TERM HEALTH OUTCOMES

EDITOR: Lorenzo Robertson

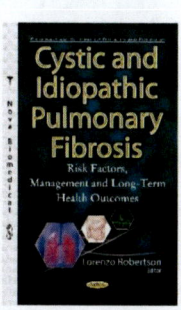

SERIES: Pulmonary and Respiratory Diseases and Disorders

BOOK DESCRIPTION: This book provides current research on risk factors of CF and IPF, as well as management options and long-term health outcomes of the disorders.

HARDCOVER ISBN: 978-1-63485-508-2
RETAIL PRICE: $160

To see a complete list of Nova publications, please visit our website at www.novapublishers.com

Related Nova Publications

NON-INVASIVE VENTILATION: A PRACTICAL HANDBOOK FOR UNDERSTANDING THE CAUSES OF TREATMENT SUCCESS AND FAILURE

EDITOR: Antonio M. Esquinas, MD, PhD

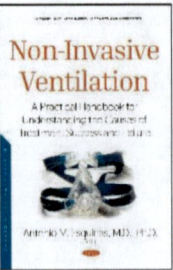

SERIES: Pulmonary and Respiratory Diseases and Disorders

BOOK DESCRIPTION: The book "Non-Invasive Ventilation: A Practical Handbook for Understanding the Causes of Treatment Success and Failure" is the first text published with well-defined objectives that analyze the success and failure response of non-invasive mechanical ventilation. Sections of this book will address different aspects of NIV ranging from perspective pathophysiological benchmarks and clinical studies, to diagnosis and monitoring elements of basic lung – patient – ventilator interaction.

HARDCOVER ISBN: 978-1-53615-199-2
RETAIL PRICE: $270

PLEURAL EFFUSIONS: CAUSES, TYPES AND TREATMENT

EDITOR: Rahul Khosla, M.D., M.B.A.

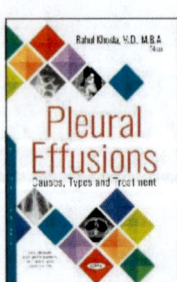

SERIES: Pulmonary and Respiratory Diseases and Disorders

BOOK DESCRIPTION: The use of point of care ultrasound, pleural manometry, and medical pleuroscopy has expanded over the last decade. The goal of writing this book was to become a source or reference for clinicians who manage patients with pleural effusions.

HARDCOVER ISBN: 978-1-53614-683-7
RETAIL PRICE: $184

To see a complete list of Nova publications, please visit our website at www.novapublishers.com